About the Author

April Rudat, MS Ed, RD, LDN is a successful breastfeeding mother of boy/girl twins. April breastfed her twins until they were two years old, and she strives to increase awareness that multiples CAN be breastfed. April passionately supports the "breast is best" philosophy; however, she also supports mothers who provide *some* breastmilk. Any breastmilk is better than no breastmilk at all.

April Rudat is a Registered Dietitian with a Master's Degree in Counseling. She is also certified in Adult Weight Management through the American Dietetic Association/ Commission on Dietetic Registration, and she has a great interest in the prevention of overweight, especially among children. In fact, to combine both of her passions, April supports the current research and encourages moms to breastfeed as a first step to obesity prevention. Visit April's websites at: www.ohyesyoucanbreastfeedtwins.com and www.dietitianapril.com.

Oh Yes You Can Breastfeed Twins!
...Plus More Tips for Simplifying Life with Twins

By April Rudat, MS Ed, RD, LDN

April Rudat, Registered Dietitian LLC

Moscow, Pennsylvania

Legal Statement

Library of Congress Control Number: 2007901753
Rudat, April.
Oh yes you can breastfeed twins! ...Plus more tips for simplifying life with twins / April Rudat.
ISBN 13: 978-0-9791549-0-4
ISBN 10: 0-9791549-0-1

Illustrations by Kristen Conniff

April Rudat, Registered Dietitian LLC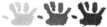

Web (book):   www.ohyesyoucanbreastfeedtwins.com
Web (practice): www.dietitianapril.com

To David and Julia, who inspired me to write this book by making breastfeeding twins look easy and by growing so beautifully on breastmilk! You've given my life so much meaning…

Contents

Part III: What I Did and What I Learned

Appendices

Preface

Based on the latest report from the Centers for Disease Control and Prevention (CDC) 128,665 sets of twins were born in 2003 (Martin et al., 2005)! Compared to 1980 when only 68,339 sets of twins were born, this increase is quite significant and appears to be growing each year. With so many more twins being born, two major issues have arisen including premature birth and low birth weight. Therefore, many mothers expecting twins want to do everything possible to create the healthiest possible outcome from the start. Along with great medical care, the best way to give your twins a great start in life is to give them breastmilk!

So you have two breasts and two babies...Perfect! You CAN breastfeed both of your babies regardless of what anyone may tell you. It is truly the best thing you can do for your twins, and it will make a huge overall difference in their lives! In this book, I will share my experiences breastfeeding twins with you, and I will also provide you with the latest research to include medical and nutrition information. I will also provide many hints, tips, and instructions to make breastfeeding and caring for your twins much simpler based on what I learned on my own journey! I will share with you what I learned the hard way so that you don't have to endure the same frustration or confusion.

I must disclose that I have not experienced breastfeeding one child (as of yet), and I am not a lactation consultant. Therefore, I provide many great references. If you are nursing one baby or want in depth lactation consultant advice, refer to my resources and suggested books (Chapter 7 – My Favorites) or contact an International Board Certified Lactation Consultant (IBCLC). However, in this book, you will find great tips for breastfeeding and maintaining your own health while breastfeeding.

I am a Registered Dietitian with a Master's Degree in Counseling, so I do know a great deal about health, mental health, and overall wellness. In fact, I do make it a point to give suggestions for your own nutrition, health, and mental health in addition to many great twin breastfeeding tips. I can also say that I am a well-seasoned breastfeeding mom of twins. I nursed my twins successfully for two years, and it paid off!

My premature twins, David and Julia, gained one to two pounds a month for the first six months (which brought them up to speed with other kids their age on the growth charts), and they were always on target for developmental milestones. Also, I have to tell you that for my twins' first nine months of life, they never got sick (even through wintertime)! Overall, they grew well, developed well, and fought off illness well! I'm obviously a huge advocate for breastfeeding twins!

In addition, I also must disclose to you that breastfeeding was my sole job for the first year of my twins' lives. I was a stay-at-home mom, so I was able to focus on breastfeeding my babies. I had a great support system, so bumps along this road weren't as tough as they could have been. Everyone's situation is different, and I truly understand this. Therefore, it is my hope that you can use at least some of the concepts in this book to make breastfeeding your twins simpler. Feel free to modify any of my concepts to meet your needs.

Please Note:

Throughout this book, I refer to babies as both "him" and "her" to remain unbiased. I also refer to your husband or partner as "spouse" for ease in reading. In addition, I interchangeably use the terms "breastfeed" and "nurse." Finally, I discuss common events and ailments in Part III ("What I Did and What I Learned") as I experienced them; however, your babies may experience these events or ailments at different times or during different ages. Use the index to obtain the page number for the issue about which you wish to learn.

Acknowledgements

Thank you so much for your support: My husband, Todd, for supporting me even though you didn't know the first thing about breastfeeding when we began this journey. You were there to support me for every moment of this entire process...from nighttime feedings to parenting confusion to diaper changes to book writing and publishing. A simple thank you does not seem like enough... My sister, Kristin Meredick Travis, who stayed with me during my tiny babies' first month of life and helped the babies to GROW by LOVING THEM SO MUCH. You did it all: From wiping a leaking breast, to changing a dozen diapers a day, to waking up at all hours of the night to hand me a baby! Mom and Dad, Nancy and John Mark Meredick, for all your "seven hour trips" to Virginia to help me and for cleaning my house despite my "control freak" tendencies! Grandma ("Baba"), Dorothy Nestor, who gave me so many breastfeeding tips from the "old school" days, who gave me support, and who gave me food in my early, high calorie days! My sister-in-law, Tara Meredick, who gave my babies SO MUCH LOVE (and preemie clothes!) and who gave me "mom" tips and breastfeeding tips for moms on the go! Shellie Sparrow, my GREAT lactation consultant, who taught me everything about breastfeeding, who got my twins to tandem breastfeed when they were less than one day old, who helped through the nipple confusion and the pacifier crisis, and who became my friend! Leslie Westman, my breastfeeding guru, nutrition activist friend, and magnificent editor, who kindly and graciously edited my book proposal and completed a pre-publication "final read" with her "eagle eye." Jeff Rudat, my brother-in-law and magnificent editor, who also kindly and graciously agreed to check out the final manuscript for a book about breastfeeding! Chantaye Johnson, my best dietitian/friend who encouraged me to breastfeed twins and who told me I COULD breastfeed twins without needing supplemental formula. Lisa Yarah, who kindly and graciously shared her touching story about providing her very premature twins with breastmilk. The Pennsylvania Registered Dietitians, who provided excellent infant and toddler food introduction tips. Kristen Conniff, my wonderfully talented artist, for your patience and your skillful and fitting illustrations and beautiful cover. Kathy Plank, my editor, who honestly and supportively helped make my manuscript into a book. Joseph Konieczny, my lawyer, who attentively and patiently provided legal guidance.

Finally, thank you to those of you who told me I could not breastfeed twins; hence, I would not have written this book to prove you wrong!

Introduction:
You Can Breastfeed Twins!

When I was four months pregnant with my twins, my sister had reconnected with a good friend, who I'll call Mary, who happened to have twin babies. Mary proceeded to tell my sister that she could not breastfeed her twins because it was too hard physically. She said she needed her rest and she just could not figure out how to get rest and breastfeed both her babies. Upon leaving the hospital, Mary was breastfeeding her babies one at a time and was truly not getting any sleep. Mary stopped breastfeeding for her own health and so that she had energy for the babies. Upon hearing all this from my sister, I hoped I could find a way to breastfeed AND stay healthy. I WOULD figure out a way...

Then when I was six months pregnant, I met a mother of eight-month-old twins, who I'll call Jane, at a meeting for my job. During the meeting introductions, I announced that I was having twins. Jane came over to me immediately at our first break, told me she had twins, and gave me 15 minutes of "twin advice." I asked her a myriad of questions, including asking her if she breastfed her babies. Jane told me that it was physically impossible and that the first six weeks of life with twins was complete hell. Again, I was feeling disheartened. But I WOULD figure out a way...

And that I did! Prior to birthing my twins, I used constant positive self-talk, telling myself that I WOULD be able to breastfeed two babies. I found my lactation consultant and picked her brain prior to my babies being born, and I did lots of reading on the subject. In addition, I notified my family and friends of my decision, and I relied upon those who were excited and supportive about my decision to breastfeed twins. Before my twins came, I was ready. And when they were born, I had all the tools in place to be successful.

In this book, I will describe all the things I did to make breastfeeding twins a success, and I will also show you through my own experience what works and what does not work. I will save you the time and energy of figuring out your own system, and I will show you that you CAN breastfeed twins!

Breastfeeding your twins is NOT physically exhausting, as long as you get rest, help from a support system, plenty of fluids, and good nutrition. You just need a good system! There are tricks, and you will learn them in this book! Also, the first six weeks of life with twins is tiring and challenging, but it is NOT hell! I loved that time with my babies and I would re-live that time again in a heartbeat.

Mary did not have a great lactation consultant and therefore lacked advice and support. She just could not figure out what to do, and she was exhausted. So she gave up. Jane thought the first weeks were hell because she didn't have enough help to breastfeed her twins simultaneously. In the meantime, she ended up spending so much time formula-feeding two tiny and hungry babies separately that she would have been able to get more rest if she breastfed her babies tandem or together! She saw no other alternatives and had no help.

In my case, I quickly deduced that you need six elements to succeed in breastfeeding twins: a great lactation consultant, plenty of rest, good nutrition, plenty of fluids, a strong support system, and motivation, especially during the challenging times.

Going into this experience, I had the nutrition knowledge to maintain my own health and thus ensure a good milk supply. I also had a great lactation consultant who even gave me her home phone number. She taught me how to breastfeed twins and got them to both breasts to feed at the same time (or *tandem*) immediately after their birth. She taught me the importance of rest and accepting help from others, and she continued to support and encourage me by returning my phone calls and emails. My husband and family also supported me both physically and emotionally, which made the first weeks a better experience.

I promise you: You can do this and survive to tell others of your success! Sure, there will be difficult times, but always remember that this is a temporary experience. The difficult times will eventually fade, and your skill will improve with each passing day! You will feel so proud that you are succeeding, and you will feel so confident that you are doing the BEST thing for your little babies. You will see tangible results with each doctor visit as weights increase, and you will notice how remarkable the babies' health is overall all because of YOUR milk. You CAN breastfeed twins! Don't let anyone say you can't! Read on for great tips for success! *Oh Yes You Can Breastfeed Twins!*

Part 1:
What You Need to Know NOW!

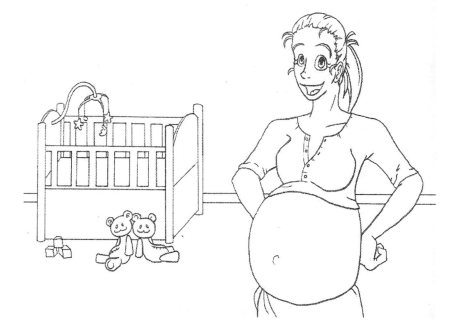

Chapter 1:
Why Breastfeed Twins?

So many people doubted that I would be able to breastfeed twins. Even at my baby shower, I told someone that I was going to breastfeed, and a family member who is a registered nurse said, "You're not going to do *that*, are you?" Other dietitians with whom I worked told me that I would probably need to supplement with formula because I "wouldn't be able to make enough milk for two babies." But I am here to say that you **can** successfully breastfeed twins. And it is the absolute best thing you can do for multiples, especially since many are born prematurely and at a low birth weight. My twins grew so rapidly and were so healthy that I knew breastfeeding was the best decision and challenge to which I've ever committed myself!

As a registered dietitian, I've learned through my studies that breastmilk is natural and superior nutritionally, which was my main reason for choosing to breastfeed twins. I also knew that breastfeeding provides so many other benefits for twins' immune systems, which is critical especially if your babies are born prematurely. I also knew that breastfed babies have fewer incidences of allergies and asthma, more skin-to-skin contact due to the frequent feedings (which I knew could possibly be linked to promoting quicker growth in infants), and an overall healthier start in life. But I won't go on and on about all the benefits of breastfeeding because chances are, if you're reading this book, you know how wonderful breastmilk is for your babies' health. (Check out Appendix A for more information on why breastfeeding is a great choice for mothers and babies.)

I will mention, however, that you will save approximately $400.00 per month (or $4,800.00 in the first year) by breastfeeding solely rather than using formula (based on the cost in the year 2006 of regular, name brand infant powder formula with iron at $13.00 per 14 oz. can assuming one can is needed per day to make 105 fl. oz. or 16-6.5 oz. bottles).

Assuming you need standard formula rather than specialized formula (in the event that your twins are premature, specialized formula will more likely be necessary) and infant size diapers (rather than preemie diapers which are more expensive), your monthly costs for formula ($400.00) and diapers ($135.00) alone would come to $535.00. Remember, this does not include the cost of additional supplies like baby wipes, medications, your health coverage co-pay times two for doctor's visits, clothing, etc. Twins can be very expensive, so you can really save some money by breastfeeding your twins full-time or even part-time!

One question that I did often ponder while nursing my twins was, "Why breastfeed *twins?*" It seems like such a difficult, daunting, and awkward task, so why do it? Well, besides the aforementioned health and nutritional benefits to your babies' immune systems and the benefit to your wallet, there are many other reasons to choose breastfeeding for your twins.

First, believe it or not, it's easy. Once you and your babies *learn* to tandem breastfeed using your breastfeeding pillow in those first couple of weeks, you will become so proficient that you will be able to enjoy a "time out" from everything else in life during breastfeeding sessions. In those early sleep deprived days, I enjoyed relaxing while nursing and felt refreshed and rested afterwards. For safety reasons, I don't recommend sleeping while nursing. However, you can safely relax, which you cannot do while trying to give each twin a bottle of formula at the same time.

This brings me to my second point: Mothers who choose to use formula don't get any down time. While nursing twins simultaneously or tandem (which is the easiest way – See Chapter 3), you have to sit and relax for 20 plus minutes, so you are forced to take a much-needed break! Mothers who formula feed their twins simultaneously don't get that break. And mothers who formula feed their twins one at a time really don't get a break!

Third, breastmilk is always ready, always sterile, always warmed to the perfect temperature, and always available (depending on how you've been taking care of yourself nutritionally – see Chapter 5.) You can do it anywhere as long as you have your breastfeeding pillow (I had three Boppies® – one for the nursery, one for the living room, and one for the car). If you want to nurse discreetly, all you need is a helper and a blanket. You don't need to pack feeding supplies besides your own large container of water...no bottles, no formula, and no sterile water needed.

Fourth, breastfeeding is very rewarding. You can see the concrete benefits from *your* breastmilk. I watched my babies gain two pounds per month every month until they were six months old, all because of my milk. I observed how other formula-fed children born around the same time as my children had so many colds, coughs, asthma, allergies, ear infections, etc. But I prevented all of this with *my* milk!

Fifth, breastfeeding two babies has the advantage of less waste. Let me explain. You have two breasts and you just had two babies. Mothers of singleton babies drip milk from the unused breast into a burp rag or some other device and that milk goes to waste. However, your milk ejection or let-down milk and subsequent release of dripping milk gets used by both babies when you feed two babies simultaneously! How resourceful!

Sixth, you may experience less engorgement in the early days of breastfeeding since you have two babies removing all that extra milk. I remember a dietitian friend of mine telling me when I was pregnant about engorgement in the early days of breastfeeding. (Engorgement is when your breasts get painfully full of milk, and your babies are best at releasing this milk.) But then she had an epiphany: She said, "You won't be nearly as engorged as women who nurse one baby since you'll have two babies to release the milk quicker!" And she was right! Since both my babies removed my milk at the same time, my engorgement was relieved more efficiently.

Seventh, you get into your pre-pregnancy jeans (the looser ones) faster than formula moms...maybe even faster than moms who are breastfeeding one baby (Heinig & Dewey, 1997)! And you don't even have to try. You will burn so many calories just by nursing twins that it's nearly impossible to eat enough. I will mention, however, that you should **not** diet. I will even be radical and say that you should not strenuously exercise until your twins are four months old so as not to dehydrate (which may decrease your milk production) and so as not to burn up any extra calories in those critical, early days of breastfeeding. Eat regularly and healthfully and enjoy some occasional splurges. And just as importantly, drink, drink, drink your water! (See Chapter 5 for nutritional recommendations for you.)

Eighth, you won't get a period for a very long time! Since your body is producing extra milk and extra lactation hormones, menstruation is further delayed (This is called *lactational amenorrhea*). In fact, I didn't get a period until after my twins' first birthday. Therefore, adding this time onto my eight months of pregnancy, I didn't have to deal with a period for almost two years! While this may sound great for period symptom removal and avoiding something that may be considered an annoyance in life, the lack of a period or amenorrhea may also reduce the risk of breast cancer since estrogen suppression during amenorrhea lowers your lifetime exposure to estrogen (Newcomb, Storer, Longnecker, Mittendorf, Greenberg, Clapp, Burke, Willett, & MacMahon, 1994).

Lastly, when you breastfeed both your babies at the same time, you can bond with both together so as not to neglect one baby during feedings. In contrast to mothers who give their twins bottles of formula one at a time, you don't have to worry about bottle-feeding one baby effectively while the other one cries for Mommy's attention. Instead, tandem nursing allows for both babies to get nutrition and attention simultaneously. It is important to spend alone time with each baby during other times throughout the day; however, feeding them together gives *both* babies attention at meal times and saves time.

At this point, let me tell you that breastfeeding my twins solely was easy because I was a stay-at-home mom. Breastfeeding was my job. If you choose to go back to work part- or full-time but wish to breastfeed your twins and use bottles of pumped breastmilk while at work, you may certainly use many of the concepts in this book. If you choose to part-breastfeed and part-formula feed your babies, your babies will still receive many of the wonderful benefits of breastfeeding. Please feel free to use some of the concepts from the book and/or modify other concepts to meet your needs.

Please know, however, that by using formula and not taking milk from your own body, you will diminish your milk supply. By not expressing your milk, you will tell your body to make less milk, thus causing a decreased milk supply. For this reason alone, I never used formula for fear of not making enough milk for my hungry babies! Every situation is unique, however, so please use whatever concepts that may help you.

Chapter 2:
Before the Twins Arrive:
What You'll Need & What You Won't

If only I had known what I am going to reveal to you in this chapter! I remember registering for my baby shower, thinking I knew what I was doing. And then I talked to some moms of infants and returned to the store to take items off my list. And then I returned to the store again to put some items back on the list. And I never registered for diapers…Good thing people bought these anyway! I could never imagine how many diapers I would need! Read on for more tips.

Your Baby Shower Registry

WHAT YOU WILL NEED:

A Nursery Made for Twins
✓ *Two cribs and two crib mattresses.*

✓ *Two crib bedding sets to include bumper pads and accessories (mobile, lamp, etc.).*

✓ *Four fitted crib sheets and four waterproof mattress pads* – Don't make the mistake of not having enough bedding! When the kids have diarrhea or vomiting episodes, you will thank yourself if you have *plenty* of extra mattress pads and sheets!

✓ *Nightlights* – You will need enough nightlights to prevent you from needing to turn on the overhead light during nighttime feedings. Enough light will also help the babies to feel safe and secure.

✓ *One or two changing tables plus multiple covers and waterproof pads for on top of the covers.*

✓ *A loveseat and a footstool.*

✓ *A recliner* – Get one that is wide enough for rocking two babies.

✓ *A full sized dresser for clothing.*

✓ *A hamper.*

✓ *Storage bins or baskets.*

✓ *Burp cloths* – These come in very handy for leaking milk, spit up, or as a quick baby tissue! Get the cotton, absorbent types, rather than the felt, over-the-shoulder types.

✓ *Two to three nursing pillows.* (I used a Boppy®, but there are also nursing pillows made just for twins.)

✓ *Nursing pillow covers* (sold at company websites or Target®).

✓ *10 + receiving blankets* – You may need to double up on these, using two at once, if your babies leave the hospital with temperature regulation issues.

✓ *Multiple blankets/quilts* – Great for the placing on the floor as play mats, for pediatric appointments when the babies need to get undressed down to their diapers, etc. (NOTE: Blankets are not needed, nor are they recommended, for the crib since they are a Sudden Infant Death Syndrome [SIDS] risk!)

✓ *Baby monitor with two + satellite monitors.*

✓ *A foot-pedal, kitchen-sized trash can with a good seal...*trust me on this one!

✓ *Antibacterial odor spray* – for your stinky trashcan.

✓ *Disinfecting wipes* for wiping the trashcan or other poop-contaminated surfaces. (But do **NOT** use these on your babies!)

✓ *A radio/CD player* – Music helps your babies to have constant noise in their environment so they are used to noise, and it also helps teach them the difference between day and night.

✓ *A steam cleaning vacuum* – The only tool to get "ground-in" puke out of a carpet!

✓ *Toys, books, rattles, teethers, and baby safe mirrors* – These should be age appropriate. Most toys are labeled by age, so follow these guidelines for safety.

✓ *Health/First Aid supplies to include:*

- *Gas drops* – I used store-brand gas drops, which have the same active ingredient and work just the same as the more expensive, name brand types.

- *Acetaminophen.* (Store-brand is fine.)

- *Ibuprofen.* (Six months or older, store brand is fine.)

- *Two soft tip thermometers* for rectal temperatures, labeled for each twin. These are great for constipation too – Ask your doctor about this first. All you do is put some petroleum jelly on the tip of the thermometer and gently insert…and out comes a poop!

- *One more thermometer* for their underarms (axillary temperatures), which can be shared.

- *One ear thermometer* for the toddler years – the armpits become much too ticklish!

- *One set of nail clippers.*

- *Two bulb syringes,* labeled for each child.

- *Baby brushes and combs.*

- *Medicine dispensers.*

- *Cool-mist humidifier* for BAD colds only. These can get moldy when used repeatedly, so be sure to clean according to package guidelines. Also, avoid "warm-mist" humidifiers as these promote mold growth faster.

- *Saline nose drops* for minor colds or crusty noses. Use separate ones for each baby.

- *Petroleum jelly.*

- *Rubbing alcohol for sterilizing.*

- *Cotton balls or gauze pads.*

- *Baby lotion or cream* for the winter months.

- *Aquaphor® cream* for chapped cheeks.

Bath Time...One Baby at a Time!

✓ *One baby bathtub with suction cups* – You can only wash one baby at a time until they have better head control. Around six months old, then they can graduate to the "big tub" with their twin and the help of a partner. Once they can sit up and you can manage them yourself, you can bathe both at once (between nine and twelve months old).

✓ *An adult-sized hand towel or washcloth* to keep the babies from sliding all over their baby tub.

✓ *One or two non-skid bath mats* for the "big" tub.

✓ *Tub spout cover* – Use the rubber types rather than the cloth types, which are easily pulled off the spout by little hands!

✓ *Baby bath wash for body and hair.*

✓ *20 washcloths* – These come in handy for bath time, and they are also useful for washing the babies' mouths when tooth buds come in and for wiping faces when you introduce solids...Just keep these face/tooth washcloths separate from bathing washcloths, which touch butts!

✓ *Eight + towels with hoods* – Having eight gives you more time between laundry days...and at about nine months old, the babies will be big enough for regular towels.

✓ *Bath toys.*

✓ *A mesh bath toy bag* with suction cups to hold toys on the wall.

For All Those Diaper Changes

✓ *A lot of wipes and diaper rash creams.* (NOTE: Baby powder is no longer recommended. Fine powder can be inhaled, leading to aspiration pneumonia.)

✓ *Preemie disposable diapers* – These diapers are for "up to 5 or 6 lbs.," so you're more than likely going to need some of these.

✓ *LOTS of "Newborn", "Size 1", and "Size 2" disposable diapers.*

✓ *A large diaper bag.*

✓ *General diaper creams* work fine for everyday use; but for very red rashes, try my favorite, *Triple Paste®*, which makes redness disappear very quickly!

Inside the Diaper Bag

✓ First off, make sure it's a *BIG* diaper bag!

✓ *12 to 20 diapers inside* – Then you won't have to refill it as often.

✓ *Two plastic wipe cases* filled to the rims with wipes. (Same here, the more you have in stock, the less refilling you'll do.)

✓ *Hand sanitizer.*

✓ *Powder-scented diaper disposal bags.*

✓ *A watch or clock.*

✓ *A pen.*

✓ *A hair tie or rubber band for you.*

✓ *Baby acetaminophen, gas drops, teething gel, sunscreen, and other medicines.*

✓ *Bulb syringes.*

✓ *Tissues* for baby boogies, your boogies, or a small spit-up.

✓ *Two onesies, two sets of pajamas, two pairs of socks, hats* (depending on the season or kind of day), *and extra outfits* (Poop happens!).

✓ *Toys/books/musical toys.*

✓ *Your large water bottle and a snack for you* (like a granola bar or dried fruit).

✓ *An oversized changing mat* – These are great as covers for those gross bathroom baby stations or for floor changing.

✓ *Pacifiers, if you use them.* Do not use them before six weeks or you can cause nipple confusion, which is REAL! If possible, stop paci's after four to six months since breaking the habit in toddlerhood is emotionally difficult. (I used them from eight weeks to three months old, when interest ended.)

✓ *A small, bendable cotton purse,* which fits your wallet and crucial necessities, can be jammed into a diaper bag easily.

✓ *Cups, spoons, bibs, food, and snacks for older babies.*

A Starter Wardrobe for Twins
✓ *10 + preemie onesies, 10 + newborn onesies, and so on* – But don't go overboard – Remember, you'll have a full load of laundry every two days or so anyway.

✓ *12 + long-sleeved, footed pajamas* (even in the summer).

✓ *Newborn skullcaps for body temperature control* (even in the summer).

✓ *Plenty of socks* (12 + pairs).

✓ *Preemie and newborn sized clothes.*

✓ *Warm car seat covers, snowsuits, and hats for winter months; light jackets for fall and spring.*

Feeding Supplies for Twins
✓ *A rented hospital pump* – Allows you to see if you will be able to do this. (I had a rented, hospital pump until my babies hit the six-week mark, then I obtained a good, electric double pump).

✓ When you realize you **can** do this, an *electric double pump with storage containers.* Many moms use the Medela® Pump in Style® or Hollister® Purely Yours® (which is the one I used). Or ask your pediatrician or other breastfeeding moms for recommendations.

✓ *Orthodontic nipple bottles* – If you need to supplement additional pumped breastmilk in the beginning or for times when you will be away from the babies. (The hospital provided me with plenty of these.)

✓ *Bottle drying rack and bottle cleaning brush.*

✓ *Dishwasher basket.*

✓ *Two infant feeding chairs.*

✓ *Two high chairs.*

✓ *Two booster feeding seats* for when you are away from home.

✓ *Six + bowls and plates with lids, six + soft spoons of varying sizes, six + toddler forks, six + infant cups* – Nuby® cups are great and feel soft like a nipple. A word on spoons: don't go for the tiny ones, as you can only use these in the very beginning of adding solids. Instead, go for a larger beginner spoon, but not so large it won't fit into the babies' mouths. Purchase spoons of varying sizes and ones with long handles for toddler use.

✓ *Bibs, bibs, and more bibs* – Remember, at about six months, you will start three meals a day which = six bibs a day. (And disposable bibs work great when you're on the run!) You can also use bibs when giving baby vitamins (since these are gross and will get spit out), so let vitamins stain the bibs rather than outfits!

✓ *"Mesh baby feeders"* – These are mesh bags that hold the real version of the baby foods that your children have already tried in jars. The kids hold these and suck the food through the mesh, which prevents choking and gives them the natural, real version of foods. Very cool to have!

✓ For older toddlers, *a small table and chair set* that is just their size.

✓ *An eating mat* for under their table – Also doubles as a great clay or arts and crafts playing mat! (You can also use an old, plastic shower curtain for this.)

On the Go with Twins

✓ *Two rear-facing infant car seats with snap-in plates plus two extra plates for another car.*

✓ *Two infant/toddler convertible seats with forward-facing and rear-facing capabilities* – These are necessary if your babies outgrow their infant seats (at 29 or more inches in length), but are not yet 20 lbs. AND one year old. Basically, these seats are for the "in between" stage, and can be used until the babies are 40 lbs.

✓ *Two 20-100 lb. forward-facing booster seats* – When the babies turn one year old AND 20 lbs, you'll need a forward-facing 20 lb.-100 lb. booster, which will last for a long while.

✓ *Car seat covers for the cold months* – GREAT in place of a bulky jacket or snowsuit!

✓ *Two car mirrors and two car sun shades* for the windows for each car.

✓ *Double stroller* – I used a front-to-back, long double stroller that fit both car seats (Graco®) rather than a wide one since the wide models tend to be difficult to use in crowded stores.

✓ *Two lightweight umbrella strollers* – For times when you have a partner and for when the babies can sit up unassisted. However, the front-to-back double stroller has better storage capacity.

✓ *Two play yards* – One regular size play yard works just fine for both babies in the beginning; however, at about six months, each baby needs their own play yard for space purposes. Two play yards are invaluable as cribs when traveling and can be placed in their storage bags and checked as luggage when traveling by air.

✓ *Small packs of disinfecting wipes* – Grocery cart handles are full of bacteria, viruses, and worse...fecal matter! Use these to wipe off the grocery cart area where your older babies will be sitting.

Other Stuff...

✓ *Two battery-operated baby swings.*

✓ *Two walkers* (with wheels taken **off** for safety) – These help strengthen your babies' trunks and help develop head control after four months old.

✓ *Two activity gyms.*

Safety Supplies

✓ *Smoke detectors* – in every room of the house. Make sure these are working on a monthly basis!

✓ *A carbon monoxide detector* in the babies' room and other locations in the house.

✓ *A radon test kit,* which can be purchased at most home stores. Check yearly. For more information, see: http://www.dep.state.pa.us/brp/Radon_Division/Radon_Homepage.htm.

✓ If you have stairs, *a staircase baby gate* – Which needs to be **screwed into** wall studs and/or banisters.

✓ *A pressure mounted gate* for the bottom of the staircase or for unsafe spaces.

✓ *Outlet covers* – lots of them!

✓ *Bite guards for the cribs* (if they don't already have them).

✓ *Shelf and bookcase clamps* to prevent tipping when the babies try to climb these (www.onestepahead.com).

✓ *Cupboard locks* (for cupboards or cabinets that hold anything unsafe: knives, cleaning supplies, etc.).

✓ *Fireplace hearth protectors, coffee table corner protectors, etc.* Or just use your **eyes** when your babies are around these surfaces, which happen to be great tools in helping them to walk! You can find just about anything in Wal-Mart®, Target®, K-Mart®, or websites like www.onesetpahead.com for safety-proofing your home!

✓ You can also rely on *tape and twisty ties* to tie up loose wires or cords, and you can tape open phone and cable jacks with regular tape to prevent tiny fingers from entering these holes!

For You!

✓ *ALWAYS WEAR A BRA!* (Or else your boobs will look like Granny's way too soon!)

- *4 + non-underwire nursing bras* – Underwire bras can cause injury to your milk ducts and can lead to a breast infection or mastitis. Trust me…I learned this one the hard way! Don't use them! I know you may want some semblance of sexiness, but it's not worth the breast pain you will endure because of underwires!

- For sleeping, I had *five sports bras* that buttoned in the front for comfort and easy access for nighttime feedings. Make sure these are not tight…Tight sports bras will have the same effect as underwire bras!

- To make life easy, you can wash your bras and breast pads with the baby laundry, which will be done more frequently than "big people" laundry. This will diminish the need for purchasing many, many more bras (due to issues like leaking or getting puke on your bra).

*Note: Only buy one or two cheap nursing bras to take to the hospital. Instead, wait until your milk comes in since you won't truly know your bra size until then. Also, I got all my nursing bras for $12.00-$15.00 each at Wal-Mart® or Target®. No need to pay $30.00 + at fancier stores. And again, AVOID UNDERWIRES!

✓ In the beginning, *ALWAYS USE NURSING PADS!*

- *One to two large boxes of disposable nursing pads* for the beginning days when you will leak a lot (Johnson & Johnson® were my favorite since they didn't stick to me.)

- *20 + cotton, washable, overnight breast pads* for overnight use and for when you are at home – These show through your bra and look like big circles on your breasts, but they are fine at home.

✓ *Lansinoh®* *nipple cream* is the best! I've used other brands, but this one is great! It's not too thick, which makes it easier to spread onto sore nipples. Be sure to use breast pads when using this bright yellow, greasy cream, or you will stain your bras!

✓ Get multiple 30 oz. (or larger) *plastic cups.* Fill a cup with some safe water, and keep pitchers of water on your nightstand and in your kitchen to keep hydrated! (See Chapter 5 on nutrition/hydration for you and Appendix B for info on safe water.)

✓ Other good *breastfeeding books.* (See my references in Chapter 7.)

✓ *Baby informational books.*

✓ *Twin, parenthood, and baby magazines.*

✓ *Two baby memory books.*

✓ *A journal* to write down funny memories, stage by stage.

✓ *Logs, forms, and charts.* (See Chapter 4.)

✓ *A notebook* for recording the twins' medical information and questions.

✓ *A calendar* for recording appointments.

✓ *A camera, video camera, and lots of photo albums* for memories of each stage...they grow SO FAST!

WHAT YOU WILL NOT NEED:

✗ *A lovely rocking chair/ottoman set* (unless you can use it as living room furniture) – These sets are wonderful for mothers who are breastfeeding one child, but there is simply not enough space to nurse two babies in these chairs unless the chair and ottoman set is the size of a recliner. A rocking recliner chair is great for rocking two babies because it is wider, and a loveseat is best for nursing two babies safely.

✗ A "diaper disposal system" or similar waste cans – You would fill these up before noon and the replacement bags aren't wallet-friendly. (You can use a regular foot-pedal, kitchen-type trashcan instead.)

✗ Cloth diapers – Are you kidding? Breastfeeding and caring for twins makes life busy enough! There is no need for another job...Sorry to those environmentally friendly folks! (Perhaps more eco-friendly diapers could be invented some day!)

✗ A bassinet – To save money, put the babies into their cribs from the beginning instead of buying two bassinets and two cribs. If your family has a shared heirloom bassinet, you would have to purchase an extra one for each additional child anyway. It's okay to forego the bassinet and use cribs from the start!

✗ Sleep positioners – These are not necessary since newborns cannot roll and will stay on their backs for many months.

✗ Stroller clips that hook two umbrella strollers together – These do not work that well, and the hooked-together strollers don't maneuver well at all. Just use a double stroller instead.

✗ Front- or back-baby carriers – Use baby carriers based on your personal preferences. In my case, I felt that it was unfair to put one baby against my chest while the other baby was in the grocery cart. If you are going to wear one while your spouse wears the other, neither baby will be left out from a nice cuddly ride. My husband and I just never used them. Instead, when shopping, we used two carts with one baby in each in their infant carriers (or later, buckled in the seatbelts). In addition, carriers are not very practical in the winter because of your coat and bulky baby snowsuits.

✗ Grocery cart protectors – While these apparatus make the point that grocery store carts are gross and full of viruses and bacteria, the simple wiping with a disinfecting wipe will accomplish the same goal for much less cash! (Grocery cart protectors run $30 to $40...multiply that by two! And are these really practical when you need to get in and out of the store quickly?)

✗ A hand pump – Must I really explain why a hand pump is ineffective?

✗ *A wipes warmer* – These are impractical when you have two poopy diapers to change as quickly as possible!

✗ *A bottle sterilizer* – For pumped milk, you can just sterilize bottles in the dishwasher or boil them before the first use. After the first use, hot, soapy water is fine for cleaning bottles.

✗ *A bottle/food warmer* – Heat *jarred baby food and cereals* based on the recommendations on the label. **NEVER nuke breastmilk.** Just put the bottle of breastmilk in a cup of warm water or serve it from the fridge! Believe it or not, babies will drink it either way.

✗ *Hand mittens for preventing scratches* – Baby nail clippers are so gentle and easy to use now that you can just keep nails short and prevent scratches on both babies.

✗ *Sleep sacks* – Are you really going to keep your babies' room so cold that you will need these? Keep the temperature comfortable, not too warm, and use footed pajamas in the winter months. Long-sleeved pajamas work great year round! Two big problems with sleep sacks: They can overheat your babies (a SIDS risk); and if they are rolling, they may get tangled in these.

✗ *A nighttime light show/musical toy* – The last thing you want to do at night is STIMULATE your twins. They'll never learn the difference between night and day with these types of toys. They look cool, but resist the temptation! Your sleep depends on it!

✗ *DVDs or videos* – The American Academy of Pediatrics (AAP) (2006) recommends **no screen time** (television, videos/DVDs, videogames, or computer time) **for children under the age of two** and no more than one to two hours of quality TV and videos a day for older children. Save DVDs for the appropriate age, and limit screen time in older kids to prevent obesity.

✗ *Nursing shirts or pajamas/nursing tank tops with "breast holes"* – These sound great, but they are not very practical. You will need both breasts exposed, so these would have to come all the way up or off anyway. Instead, use form-fitting shirts that can be lifted up and will stay up or strappy tank tops (even under sweaters) so that straps can be taken down.

And remember: Keep all store receipts so you can return unwanted items!

Chapter 3:
Creating a Nursery Environment Conducive to Breastfeeding Twins

Regarding your nursery, I just want to expand on a few of my aforementioned "What You Will Need" items. Many of these items serve to create a nursery environment conducive to breastfeeding twins. Here, I will provide instructions and illustrations to make breastfeeding twins a simpler concept for you.

The Physical Environment

The Loveseat
As mentioned earlier, the rocker chairs with a matching ottoman are really pretty and comfortable for one person, but these are not very practical for nursing twins. You simply will not fit in this chair with your nursing pillow and two babies. I started off with a regular recliner chair. It worked beautifully for nursing the babies since my sister stayed the first month after their birth and could hand me one baby at every feeding. However, once she left my home, I had no way of fetching both babies and getting them onto my nursing pillow safely.

I discovered that a *loveseat* was the best device for nursing my twins. Since a recliner is larger in width, you can use a rocking recliner in a nearby room to rock your babies as needed. However, I recommend using a *loveseat* for breastfeeding from the start since a loveseat is much larger and thereby easier for getting two babies to your breasts. I wish I had done this from the start! Here is the protocol for breastfeeding twins using a loveseat:

1. Place a comfortable loveseat in the nursery before your twins are born. It doesn't have to be new, but it needs to be comfortable. In fact, an old loveseat is better since it may get puked or pooped on.

2. Put the quilt from your baby set onto the loveseat to protect it from spit-up, poop, etc. and to display it since you should not use this quilt in the crib (placing items in the crib that are soft or plush, including blankets and quilts, can lead to Sudden Infant Death Syndrome - SIDS).

3. Place a pillow in the center of the loveseat for back ergonomics.

4. Get a pretty footstool and place this where your feet will need to rest. Placing your feet on a footstool not only helps support your back by creating good posture, but it also helps keep the babies' heads higher than their bodies since your knees will be raised. Keeping the babies' heads higher than their bodies can prevent reflux symptoms and fluid from getting into their Eustachian tubes of their ears (a cause of ear infections).

YOUR LOVESEAT & SUPPLIES:
BACK PILLOW, FOOTSTOOL, & NURSING PILLOW

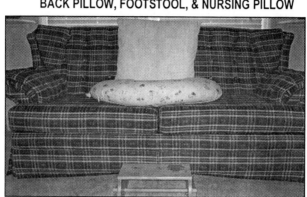

To Begin...
First and foremost, I have discovered the following technique to be the safest when attempting to get two babies from cribs to breast without a helper. I am simply providing this technique as a suggestion.

DISCLAIMER: Use this technique at your own risk, and use it with caution. This is not medical advice; it is merely a suggestion. Consult your pediatrician and/or lactation consultant first about techniques to get two babies to your breasts for breastfeeding.

1. When under four months old (or before rolling begins), to fetch my twins for a feeding, I grabbed baby A and placed him lying flat on the appropriate side of the loveseat (the side of the breast that was his for this particular feeding) with his head towards the **back** of the loveseat.

2. Then, I retrieved baby B and placed her on the other side of the loveseat in the same manner.

3. While doing this, I NEVER TOOK MY EYES OFF MY BABIES!!

MY BABIES' POSITIONING ON THE LOVESEAT WHEN
YOUNGER THAN FOUR MONTHS OLD (BEFORE THEY COULD ROLL):

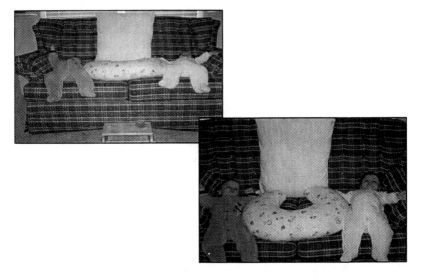

4. Sit down in the middle of the loveseat against your back pillow, grab your nursing pillow, and grab the fussier baby first, placing her onto the nursing pillow in a football hold position.

5. Proceed to grab your other twin in a football hold on the other side, and you will be set to nurse! (See photos below of correct baby placement onto loveseat and of football hold. Both babies should be resting on each side of the nursing pillow, lying on their sides.)

HERE'S YOUR LOVESEAT – YOU SIT WITH YOUR BACK AGAINST THE PILLOW:

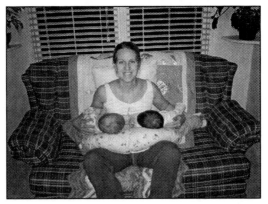

TANDEM BREASTFEED ALL THE TIME TO SAVE ON TIME!

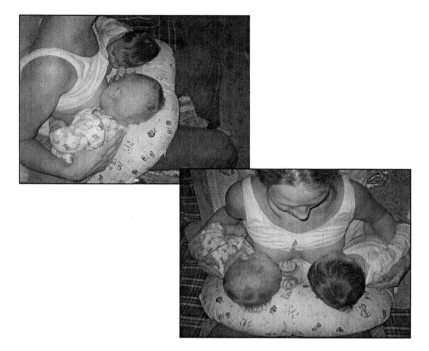

Never place your babies' heads towards the edge of the loveseat, as they will use their legs to push themselves off. Just the same, never sit your babies upright in the corners of the loveseat. They will fall off. It's best to use the aforementioned technique with an extremely watchful eye on both babies as you sit down. Or place the less active baby down first, and hold the active baby as you sit. Then you can place the active baby directly on your nursing pillow first, and reach over and grab the baby on the couch second. One other safety recommendation is to place pillows on the floor in the event of an accidental fall.

NOTE: NEVER PLACE YOUR
BABIES HEADS AT THE EDGE OF
THE LOVESEAT AND NEVER LET
YOUR BABIES SIT UPRIGHT ON
THE LOVESEAT (SEE RIGHT)!
THEY WILL FALL!

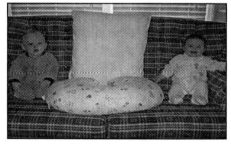

THIS IS NOT SAFE!

When my babies were older than four months, I found it safer to grab one baby and place him on the floor next to the loveseat. Then, I got the other baby. I placed each baby onto my nursing pillow one at a time and began nursing. Once my babies started crawling, however, I had to adjust my technique since they would crawl away. And once they started standing in their cribs, I was able to pick them both up at once and then carry them together to the loveseat for breastfeeding.

Your Room, Their Own Room, Or Separate Rooms?
The answer to this question is totally up to you; however, consider the following thoughts. Many breastfeeding mothers want their babies close and therefore in their room, but this would require getting a loveseat and cribs for both babies into the master bedroom! My personal belief is that the babies can keep each other company in their own room from the start, and the baby monitor can keep you connected to the babies and their cries or sounds very well. In addition, putting them in their own room together from the start will also prevent a very difficult transition from "mom and dad's room" to the nursery as the babies' bedroom.

In addition, never, **NEVER** let your babies sleep in your bed. This can lead to death by suffocation by either you or your spouse or from your bedding. Even allowing a baby to sleep on your chest during your nighttime sleep or daytime naps *can lead to death*. Also, having older kids in bed with you and your spouse is really never a good idea since it can lead to a long-term bad habit...one which can lessen quality evening time with your spouse and decrease any sex life you may have left! And remember, it is easier not to begin a habit at all than to work on breaking one...

My opinion is to let the babies sleep in their own, *shared* room. I very emphatically do not agree with separate bedrooms for multiples. Your twins spent nine months (hopefully) together in very close quarters in the womb; therefore, it is only natural to continue to keep them close together. Parents may wonder about the babies waking each other with their cries, but I can attest that a phenomenon exists whereby they do not wake one another. Or, if they do startle one another with their cries initially, they will soon get used to each other's noises and learn to ignore the cries. In my case, this phenomenon existed until my babies were toddlers!

Although my babies are just toddlers now as I write this book, I plan on keeping my twins in the same room until they verbally request their own rooms. In my opinion, it is imperative that parents be "child centered" in regard to keeping your babies together. Let them tell you when they are ready to individuate and get their own bedroom.

One or Two Cribs?
Although many pediatricians recommend keeping twins together in the same crib to promote warmth, a sense of safety and security, and growth, the American Academy of Pediatrics (AAP) does not address putting multiples together into one crib. Generally speaking, the AAP and other groups deem it unsafe for babies to co-sleep or co-bed with other adults or children because of the risk of suffocation, entanglement, and/or SIDS. In addition, there are not enough randomized, controlled trials to determine if it is a safe choice to place multiple babies in one crib (Witt, 2006).

The dangers of co-bedding include overheating and entanglement with each other or with bedclothes (Witt, 2006). Therefore, a potential solution to prevent the possible complications of co-bedding in one crib is to use two cribs in the nursery, placed against or very close to one another. This possible solution will allow your babies to remain in very close proximity in a safe manner. You can put the cribs against one another so that the babies can touch hands and see one another through the crib slats. With this suggestion, the babies will still be able to maintain closeness in a safer way.

Other Supplies
I had one changing table upstairs and one downstairs. Changing tables really save your back, and you definitely need diapers stored around the house since you never know when a diaper will reach its storage capacity and blow out. Remember: not all diapers are created equal. I splurged on the name brand diapers rather than dealing with throwing away clothing when diapers malfunctioned! As for wipes, I found Wal-Mart's® generic store brand wipes (the unscented variety) to be as good as the more expensive, name brand ones.

As for a dresser, I used an adult-sized version since it could fit clothing and supplies for two little people. I also used a room with a walk-in closet for my nursery for storing baby supplies and clothing. A walk-in closet is nice, but is not necessary – a big closet will do just fine. I also had another entire room in my home designated as a playroom for the supplies that seem to multiply overnight—two walkers (with wheels removed), two infant feeding chairs, two car seats, two high chairs, baby gyms, baby toys, and baby books. Speaking of books, please use caution with bookshelves since many toddlers try to scale them like mountain climbers. Bolt these to the wall to reduce the risk of falls or death. You can find products to mount them to the wall at: www.onestepahead.com.

Finally, I want to mention nightlights and trashcans. A good, bright nightlight (or two or three) can prevent the need to turn on the overhead light for overnight feedings and diaper changes. This is critical for creating the differentiation of "day" versus "night" (See next page). Invest in as many as you need to achieve this goal. The dusk to dawn nightlights are great. As for trashcans, pay the $50.00 (or so) for a kitchen-sized, foot pedal trashcan with a good seal. The "diaper disposal system" concept is wonderful, but these will not hold twin quantities of diapers. "Diaper disposal systems" also conveniently require their own bags, which may hurt your wallet. You can find good foot pedal trashcans with good seals at K-Mart®, Wal-Mart®, Target®, or other home stores.

An Environment for Sleeping

In your nursery, create an environment of "day" versus "night." For your own good night's rest, from day one, you must teach your babies "day" versus "night" by turning the lights on and opening the blinds in the room during all *day* hours. In addition, when it became day, I turned on the radio and left it at a reasonable volume all day long. I truly believe that music helps calm you, the Mommy, as well, which can help your milk to eject more effectively and keep your stress level at bay. To recap, *day* includes a bright room and music (country music in our home) all day long *including* during nap times. I can attest that this works! Babies do not need a dark, quiet room and a quiet house for naptimes!

 Nighttime was drastically different from day in that we turned off the radio, shut the blinds, and put away all the toys and books. My husband and I talked quietly, changed both sets of diapers, and got both babies into their pajamas. I would then nurse the kids, and my husband would leave the room quietly. He would return in 10 to 15 minutes to burp the babies, and he would stay until they became ready for bed. They became ready for bed when they fell asleep at the breast (in those early days when they were tiny, sleepy babies) or when they stopped nursing for longer than five minutes.

 And I have to tell you that from day one until the present, I needed a helper to get both babies down in their cribs at bedtime. While sitting on the loveseat, I had both babies lying on the nursing pillow, so I essentially did not have enough arms to get them both safely to their cribs. I could have put one baby on the floor in order to get the other baby to bed, but then the baby on the floor would have an emotional meltdown. This would cause the baby in my arms to become frustrated and angry as well, making bedtime a loud and crazy experience. Therefore, when my husband traveled on business or when I would be alone for bedtime, I had a family member or friend come over to help put the babies down.

 I want to disclose one more important fact about day versus night. *You* create "day" and you create "night" by your behavior and setting changes. For example, if I was feeling run down from a rough night of hungry babies, I didn't make it "day" until 10:30 or 11:00 am. I left the twins in their cribs to "sleep in" and delayed the start of day (blinds opened, radio on, activity, etc.). They seemed to appreciate the extra sleep as well and learned the difference between day and night by my behaviors and environmental cues.

Setting a Bedtime
As far as bedtime goes, I wholeheartedly believe in setting a bedtime that suits your babies *and* you, the parents. (Many parents set a bedtime based on their children's needs alone.) Yes, you do need to watch for your twins' tiredness cues; however, don't put your children to bed at 7:00 pm if you don't want to wake at 5:00 am or earlier. The bedtime you initiate soon after their birth will stick; so pick a bedtime that works for everyone.

My husband and I chose the 8:00 to 9:00 pm timeframe as a bedtime. As mentioned, in the early days, I "initiated day" later (10:30 am or so) to catch up on some needed sleep. When the twins started sleeping through the night at five months old, however, they still went to bed at 9:00 pm and slept until 8:30 or 9:00 am the next morning. As a stay-at-home-mom, this was great! I never felt so refreshed! And the twins were happy too.

Around 10 months, however, the twins started wanting to go to bed earlier. In fact, they probably would have liked a 7:00 pm bedtime. In reaction to their new tiredness cues, I changed bedtime to 8:00. This worked for everyone in that they still slept until 8:00 am the next morning (not waking too early), and they went down to sleep better since they were not overtired.

In essence, shape your babies' bedtimes to fit your routine, but collaborate with them based on their tiredness cues (becoming fussy, defiant, rubbing eyes, yawning, etc.). An overtired baby will give you a hard time going to sleep; therefore, work together to choose the best bedtime.

An Environment with Routine

Develop a *routine*, but not a schedule. A schedule is rigid and is set by times, so a schedule will not work with twins since you have two individual (and different) babies for which to care. A routine, on the other hand, includes a series of events happening in the same order through your babies' day. A routine is comforting to babies, making them feel safe and secure in knowing what to expect and what will happen next in their typical day. Babies who have a routine, therefore, may be less likely to act out or fuss since they know in what order things happen.

I will say, however, that I do not endorse a strict routine. For example, if a relative's birthday party falls during naptime or runs into bedtime, it is not healthy to skip the party to retain the routine. In life, we all have routines, and we all have things that may disrupt our routines. We adjust, and the babies need to learn this as well. Therefore, the best way to teach your babies the concept of adjusting is to allow for breaks in routine for special occasions. Then, return to the basic routine the next day.

A few words about setting "schedules": It is especially important **not** to set a schedule of nursing times (unless your babies are premature and need to be awakened every three hours to feed in their early days of life). It is of utmost importance to feed your babies on demand *and* together. Feeding on demand (when babies show cues that they want to eat: rooting, grasping, mouthing, salivating, etc.) will keep your milk supply up and will help your babies to grow most effectively. Feeding on demand may be every two to three hours, but it may be even sooner during growth spurts. (Feeding every two hours starts from the time you start to feed; therefore, you are essentially feeding them one and a half hours after the last feed.) Feed on demand for the best milk supply possible! Remember, it is challenging to feed on demand, but it is only for a short period of time in your life. You will get through it!

I also highly recommend feeding your twins **simultaneously or tandem all the time** using a double football hold. (NOTE: You may find another position that works for you.) This is critical advice that I learned the hard way. In the beginning during nighttime feedings when one baby would wake, I thought, "Oh, my son is sleeping so nicely. I'll just feed my daughter." And then 15 minutes after I would return to bed at 3:30 am, my son would wake up screaming, wanting to nurse. I was essentially awake during all evening hours, which caused me to feel run down and useless to my babies. It was then that I decided to feed the babies at the same time *every time.*

If one baby awakened and wanted to nurse, I would wake the other baby and feed them together. It sounds cruel, but there simply are not enough hours in the day to feed your babies separately and remain a healthy and sane person. You have to take care of yourself or you will be useless to your babies both physically and emotionally. Feeling too run down will cause you to fail. Succeed by nursing your twins simultaneously!

The double football hold was the only nursing position that worked for me. I used the same position every time, but I alternated which baby got which breast at every feeding to even out breastmilk transfer (and my breasts!). Every other position was awkward or even dangerous. And once the babies became more active on my nursing pillow at about six months, the double football hold proved to be the safest and best position for my entire time breastfeeding twins.

What about assigning one baby to one breast? It sounded like a good and less confusing solution to me until I found out that each baby suckles differently and takes different amounts of milk. To keep both breasts producing adequate milk and to keep both breasts the same size (for aesthetic purposes), alternate breasts for *each feeding* instead.

For example:

✓ FIRST FEEDING: Baby A gets RIGHT breast/ Baby B gets LEFT breast.
✓ NEXT FEEDING: Baby A gets LEFT/ Baby B gets RIGHT.
✓ And so on for all feedings...
✓ See Chapter 4 for "Feeding Logs." Use these to record who gets which breast at which feeding to keep milk transfer even. Keep feeding logs in the babies' room on a clipboard, and take them with you when you're out.

Personal Values
Add your personal values to your routine as well. If you pray or meditate, do so with your babies to teach them your personal values. Make reading books to your babies part of your routine *every day.* I also played country music all day long (which helped make it "day" versus "night"), and I truly believe this music helped my state of mind as well since it prevented my home from becoming silent and lonely. In addition, the music got the babies used to noise. Therefore, I did not have to tiptoe around during the day to prevent them from waking up. I could actually clean the entire house during naptimes, and the babies wouldn't wake from my cleaning noises!

In general, I made sure that my babies experienced these five elements daily:

1. Spiritual development (if applicable) – by praying/meditating together every morning (And who knows? Maybe they will be able to memorize prayers easier and more readily!)

2. Physical activity – could include going for walks in the stroller as well as tummy time, floor time, rolling/crawling/creeping/standing time, dancing, playing, etc. Also includes time outdoors (whether out shopping, out playing in the grass, or out for a stroll).

3. Socialization – by getting the babies out of the house and around other people, by allowing the babies to play with other children of varying ages, and by giving your babies time with other family members and friends to create bonds with others besides mom and dad.

4. Emotional wellness – includes giving lots of encouragement, "I love you's", kisses and hugs, positive reinforcement, skin-to-skin contact, and looking into their eyes when speaking to them. Also includes saying each baby's name when addressing him or her, using their names when feeding, and using manners and respect when speaking to the babies (including saying "please," "thank you," and "may I").

5. Intellectual development – reading many books daily, talking to the babies regularly, answering the babies when they're babbling, teaching them the names for things/people/body parts, and singing to them daily.

An Example of Routine

To develop a routine, follow your babies' leads. They will let you know when they are tired, hungry, or active. A routine may include something like this for newborn twins:

✓   In the morning, wake up, nurse for 20 to 45 minutes, sleep for 2 ½ hours.
✓   Wake up, nurse for 20 to 45 minutes, play for 15 minutes, sleep for 1 ½ hours.
✓   Wake up, nurse for 20 to 45 minutes, get a bath, sleep for an hour.
✓   Wake up, nurse for 20 to 45 minutes, play for 30 minutes and read books, sleep for an hour.
✓   Wake up, nurse for 20 to 45 minutes, play for 30 minutes, sleep for an hour.
✓   At night, wake up, nurse for 20 to 45 minutes, sleep for 2 ½ hours.
✓   Wake up, nurse for 20 to 45 minutes, sleep for 2 ½ hours.
✓   Wake up, nurse for 20 to 45 minutes, sleep for 2 ½ hours.

On the other hand, a routine for six-month-old twins may look something like this:

✓   Sleep through night, wake up, nurse for 15 minutes, play for 10 minutes, eat breakfast cereal.
✓   Nap for 1 ½ to 2 hours, wake up, nurse for 10 minutes, eat lunch cereal, get baths.
✓   Nap for 2 hours, nurse for 10 minutes, play for one hour.
✓   One baby sleeps for 20 minutes while the other plays, play for one hour and read books, nurse for 20 minutes.
✓   Play for 2 hours, nurse for 7 minutes, eat dinner meal.
✓   Play for an hour, nurse for 15 to 20 minutes, go to bed for the night.

Additional Tips For Mom

Find ways to *sleep*. In my case, I extended "night" so that I could essentially sleep in until 11:00 am since I was up all night long (every two to three hours) for feedings. With two very different babies, I couldn't nap during the day; so sleeping in really worked well for me. In fact, a lot of people tell you when you are pregnant to "sleep when the baby sleeps." However, you have TWO babies. And two individual newborns are not always going to want to take naps at the same time, leaving you napless. Instead, find a way to sleep in. And foster that "day" versus "night" difference and the same routine for your babies. Before you know it, they will be sleeping through the night and taking naps at the same time! (For me, this happened at four and a half months.)

From day one, keep *good posture*! This is so important! At about five months old, my babies became a bit stronger and a bit squirmier during feedings. I found myself contorting my back to meet their comfort needs. At this time, I also started solids. In turn, I found myself slouching while feeding them their solids. I also began a terrible habit of bending at my waist to pick them both up. And before I knew it, my back was a sore mess! Making good posture a priority eventually led to diminished back pain! (One great way to alleviate your back pain is to ask that good old spouse of yours for a massage at the end of the day. You deserve it!)

Make it a priority to get some "*me*" time. Especially if you are a stay-at-home-mom, you need some time to do things YOU enjoy. This also helps you to maintain your identity rather than only feeling like "mommy" or "wife." You are a beautiful, strong, and special woman, and you deserve to preserve some of your interests and passions.

For me, I took time during every nap to write. Writing has always been a passion of mine, so I ended up writing this book during naps alone! Yes, sometimes the laundry piled up and sometimes the dishes stayed dirty until 3:00 pm, but I took the time to write as often as possible to unwind and express my creative self.

Take the time to do something that you enjoyed pre-pregnancy or something you have wanted to do for a long time. Do this during naptime or after the babies have gone to sleep for the night. Or better yet, ask your spouse to "baby sit" for an hour or two while you catch up on some quality time with yourself!

Chapter 4:
Keeping Track: Forms, Logs, & Charts

I will warn you: The following information may sound tedious. You have two babies to care for, and now I'm recommending that you keep track of all sorts of stuff! But forms, logs, and charts will actually make your life simpler because they will help you keep track of your children's medical issues, feedings, who got which breast last, and diaper content! And you can decide what will work for your situation, choosing only those forms that are applicable to you!

First, I will explain each form/log/chart and how I used it. Then, I will give you a sample of each form that you may use for your own benefit. The forms/logs/charts are as follows:

A Pretty Journal

Record important and cute events on a monthly (or more often) basis for the twins to read when they are older or for you to use as a reference for milestones. I had separate journals including a pregnancy journal and then a birth through one-year old journal and so on.

A Medical Notebook

Use a notebook to record all your babies' medical information. Record the following:

✓ Every appointment date and what happened at that appointment.

✓ Weights, lengths, head circumferences.

✓ Vaccines given. (Or you can use a vaccine record.)

✓ Illnesses and issues that came up at the visit.

✓ Also write questions that you may want to ask the doctor in this book as they come up, because otherwise, you will forget the question by the time you get to your next appointment. You have too many other things to remember!

A Calendar

A small or purse-sized calendar for the babies' appointments, events, and food schedule (see below) is a must to keep everything straight! Then, you can bring this to each appointment to make future appointments. Also, put your information/appointments on here so that you know what days are occupied.

A sample calendar page at 5 ½ months old when I started solids *

November						
Sunday	Monday	Tuesday	Wednesday	Thursday	Friday	Saturday
		1 rice cereal	2 rice cereal	3 rice cereal	4 rice cereal	5 rice cereal
6 rice cereal	7 rice cereal	8 barley cereal	9 barley cereal	10 barley cereal	11 barley cereal	12 barley cereal
13 barley cereal	14 barley cereal	15 oatmeal	16 oatmeal	17 oatmeal	18 oatmeal	19 oatmeal
20 oatmeal	21 oatmeal	22 squash	23 squash	24 squash	25 squash	26 carrots – reaction(D)
27 squash	28 sweet potatoes	29 sweet potatoes	30 sweet potatoes			

*See Appendix B for more nutrition information

The Feeding/Diaper Log

Use this very important log to record daily feedings. On a feeding log, you can record feeding times, which baby got which breast, how long the feeding was (**optional), how much supplemental breastmilk in a bottle they got (if needed; see more on supplementation in Chapters 15-16), and contents of the diaper at that feeding. I used these logs (see the next few pages) for the whole first year! It just helped to keep everything straight!

** NOTE: It is more important to make sure the babies are latched and suckling well. Watch them and their suckling instead of watching the clock! Listen for a slowing in swallows and a change in behaviors to know when the feeding is over. "Tune in" to your babies' feeding habits, not the clock!

Example: My Feeding/Diaper Log with Space for Supplemental Breastmilk

*NOTE: This was useful when my twins were newborns, needing extra, fortified breastmilk via a bottle and needing to be awakened for feedings. I **DO NOT** endorse setting a feeding schedule **or** supplementing with a bottle of formula (unless your physician recommends this). Breastfeed on demand for best success!

Date / Times	Name of Baby	Breast Side	Time Spent (min.) (optional)	Bottle (cc)	Diaper Content
6/15/05					
Midnight	David	R	25	20	Pee
	Julia	L	25	30	Pee
3:00	David	L	25	22	Pee, poop
	Julia	R	20	30	Pee
6:00	David	R	20	17	Pee
	Julia	L	20	30	Pee, poop
9:00	David	L	25	15	Pee, poop
	Julia	R	20	30	Pee, poop
Noon	David	R	35	25	Pee, poop
	Julia	L	30	30	Pee, poop
3:00	David	L	45	22	Pee
	Julia	R	40	30	Pee, poop
6:00	David	R	30	20	Pee, poop
	Julia	L	30	30	Pee
9:00	David	L	50	15	Pee
	Julia	R	45	30	Pee

Your Copy: Feeding/Diaper Log with Space for Supplemental Breastmilk
You may copy this page for your use.

Date / Times	Name of Baby	Breast Side	Time Spent (optional)	Bottle (cc)	Diaper Content

Example: My Feeding/Diaper Log
When the Babies No Longer Needed a Bottle

Date / Times	Name of Baby	Breast side	Time Spent (min.) (optional)	Diaper Content
12/27/05				
9:08 am	David	L	20	Pee, poop
	Julia	R	20	Pee, poop
1:15 pm	David	R	15	Pee
	Julia	L	10	Pee
3:40 pm	David	L	10	Pee, poop
	Julia	R	10	Pee, poop
5:58 pm	David	R	25	Pee
	Julia	L	25	Pee
7:30 pm	David	L	10	Pee, poop
	Julia	R	7	Pee
9:14 pm	David	R	20	Pee
	Julia	L	20	Pee
----	David			
	Julia			
----	David			
	Julia			

Blank Copy: Feeding/Diaper Log
You may copy this page for your use.

Date / Times	Name of Baby	Breast side	Time Spent (optional)	Diaper Content

Growth Charts

As of April 2006, the World Health Organization (WHO) released "Child Growth Standards" growth charts that are representative of all countries and suitable for both breastfed and formula fed babies (WHO, 2006). In the past, the Centers for Disease Control and Prevention's (CDC) growth charts were the official growth charts; however, these charts are mainly based on formula fed babies (AAP, 2004). Therefore, the new WHO growth charts are more representative for your breastfed babies.

In fact, WHO states that their charts represent "how children should grow" based on the best current health recommendations including "all women breastfeeding, obtaining standard pediatric care for their children, and not smoking" (WHO, 2006). Breastfeeding is made the biological "norm" for these charts, and WHO determined that the breastfed infant **should be** the normative growth model for a chart (WHO, 2006).

Growth charts allow you to track your babies' growth compared to other infants their age. Two points to remember: First, many pediatric offices still use the CDC's growth charts, which are only appropriate for formula-fed babies (who tend to weigh more than breastfed babies, especially during the six to 12 month range when most moms stop breastfeeding) (AAP, 2004).

If plotted on a CDC curve, it's more important that your babies follow an upward trend on the curve, rather than being at the 50th percentile, per say. Or, you can simply visit: http://www.who.int/childgrowth/standards/en/ for the new WHO growth charts. Just be sure to click on the "Birth to 5 Years" **PERCENTILES** charts so these are comparable to other charts and easy to understand. Print and bring copies of these to the pediatrician's office for use in your babies' charts, or keep your own records on these forms.

Second, some physicians may use the babies' *corrected age*, which is a formula used to adjust the babies' ages based on their gestational age and current age if they were born prematurely. Ask your physician if nurses are using your babies' actual age or corrected age on the growth curve. (Corrected age is calculated by subtracting the number of weeks of prematurity from the birth age.)

As mentioned, you can obtain online copies of the WHO Child Growth Standards charts at: http://www.who.int/childgrowth/standards/en/. There are separate growth charts for boys and girls and for weight for age, length for age, and Body Mass Index (BMI) for age. Remember; use **percentiles** for comparability to the CDC versions (instead of using z-scores). Please note that these growth charts use kilograms (kg) instead of pounds (lbs.) and centimeters (cm) instead of inches (in.). At pediatrician visits, simply ask the nurse to give you the babies' heights and weights in both pounds and kilograms as well as in inches and centimeters. They can do this easily!

If you need to convert pounds (lbs.) and inches (in.) to kilograms (kg) and centimeters (cm), use the following equations:

Weight

✓ $kg = \dfrac{lbs.}{2.2}$

If you have lbs. and oz. for your babies' weights, do the following math:

✓   (16 oz. **x** the number of lbs.) **+** the number of oz.

✓   Take this total **/** 16 and then **/** 2.2 **= your baby's weight in kg**

* If your babies weights are in grams (g):

✓   1 kg = 1000 g

✓   To get kg, take g **/** 1000 = **kg**

✓   To get lbs., take kg **x** 2.2 = **lbs.**

Length

✓   cm = in. **x** 2.54

Body Mass Index (BMI)

✓   BMI = weight in lbs. **x** 703 **/** height in inches **/** height in inches

**Or just ask the nurse or pediatrician to
complete these calculations for you!**

Chapter 5:
How to Breastfeed Twins Successfully

In my experience, I have found that there are seven steps to breastfeeding twins successfully:

1. Find a Great Lactation Consultant
2. Rest and Relax
3. Eat Well to Make Good Quality Milk
4. Stay Hydrated for Good Quantities of Milk
5. Nurse Often, Pump Wisely, and NEVER Use Formula
6. Get a Good Support System and Ask Them for Help
7. Stay Motivated

Read on to learn more about these steps!

1. Find a Great Lactation Consultant

I was lucky. I met my great lactation consultant prior to delivery. My lactation consultant, Shellie, was also the teacher for my childbirth education classes, so I picked her brain after every class about breastfeeding twins. She told me that I absolutely could breastfeed twins and make plenty of milk for both babies. Shellie also told me to ask for her at the time of my delivery so that she could get the twins to breastfeed tandem or simultaneously soon after birth so I could learn the twin breastfeeding mechanics prior to being discharged from the hospital.

My twins were born prematurely at 34 weeks gestation, but they were generally in good health. To be expected, immediately after birth, my babies were whisked away for tests. Soon after I got to my room, one of my nurses told me that my babies had to be being given formula because they needed nutrition to gain weight quickly. She said that although it's very valuable and that the babies need it, I only had colostrum, (the protein-rich pre-milk or "liquid gold" produced during the first two to three days after birth that is only released in small quantities). She said my milk wouldn't come in for at least two days, meaning that I would only make drops of colostrum until my milk came in full force. My babies simply needed more nutrition than what I had at the time.

What did I do? I asked for a breast pump and a lactation consultant. It was my goal to get my milk in as quickly as physiologically possible. In the meantime, a wacky lactation consultant came in with a single breast pump and a syringe for feeding colostrum to the twins. A single breast pump?! What?? I had two babies and two breasts, so why couldn't I get a double pump?

And then she made me very nervous with the syringe feedings (which are supplemental feedings where you squirt colostrum or breastmilk into babies' cheeks through a small syringe rather than using a bottle, which can cause nipple confusion – See Chapter 10 for more on nipple confusion). This lactation consultant never even told me about bottles with orthodontic nipples, which are so much easier for supplemental milk, and she thought pumping one breast would do for twins!

I waited for Shellie to come in for her shift. She gave me another breast pump attachment so I could pump both my breasts at the same time, get my milk in faster, and get the nurses to stop giving formula. She also brought my babies from the nursery to my room so that we could get them to latch on successfully ASAP. Within the first 24 hours of life, Shellie had both babies at both breasts tandem nursing! She also showed me how to do this myself using a nursing pillow. Soon enough, my milk came in and she showed me where to take it in the nursery so that my babies received supplemental breastmilk rather than supplemental formula, and she also taught me about the human milk fortifier that was being put into my milk to make it higher in calories.

Shellie gave me her home phone number and email address, and I called and emailed her many times until the babies were three months old. Now I send her Holiday cards! She has become a good friend, and she repeatedly told me how I was doing the best possible thing for my babies by breastfeeding. My advice to you:

✓ Find a great lactation consultant well before your babies are born. She should be more than willing to teach you how to breastfeed twins, and she should have a patient and helpful attitude. Like any profession, not all lactation consultants are great. Find one that works for you! Ask for her phone number, pager number, and email address. If she refuses, she's not the one for you. You have special needs with twins and will need extra help!

✓ Make sure your lactation consultant teaches you how to breastfeed successfully *before* your hospital discharge. This includes getting both babies to latch properly and getting both babies to breastfeed tandem or at the same time.

✓ If you are having latching issues, make an appointment for additional help. Some lactation consultants even come to your home! If you need a supplemental nutrition system (a bottle of breastmilk with attached tubes that are taped to your breasts to provide additional milk) or other types of feedings (syringe, cup, spoon, or finger feedings), make sure you are very proficient before you leave the hospital!

✓ Once the babies are born, demand a double-sided breast pump and pump after every feeding to get your milk to come in (usually every two to three hours, eight to ten times a day). Even if you make 2 cc (30 cc = 30 mL = one ounce), save it and take it to the fridge in the nursery!

✓ **Immediately** rent a pump or purchase one (See my suggestions in Chapter 2) as soon as you can so you have it for your day of discharge from the hospital. (Your babies may have to stay in the hospital longer than you, so get a pump fast!)

✓ Drink to thirst and eat well to make quantity and quality milk (read on!).

✓ Get your rest and get your babies on both breasts for every feeding. My babies stayed an extra week in the hospital, and I went to the hospital for each daytime feeding and all but one nighttime feeding to keep my milk supply up. I also pumped after every feeding at home. For the night feedings I missed, I pumped for 15 minutes, stored the milk in the fridge, and took it to the hospital for my babies.

About latching on:

✓ Get your lactation consultant to help you get both your babies latched on properly.

✓ Moms with one baby get to use two hands to promote a latch (a latch is the proper position of the baby's mouth around the nipple). They use one hand to hold the baby and the other hand to hold or cup their breast. You cannot do this. You need one hand to hold each baby, which leaves no hand to do the breast cupping. Make sure your lactation consultant teaches you to get your babies to latch using only one hand while you are still in the hospital!

✓ Your babies should take in both your nipple and the surrounding area, the areola. You need your babies to open their mouths wide to take in this big area. They can do this...trust me! My three-pound babies did! Sometimes you can accomplish this very easily by getting your breast into their mouths during a yawn or big cry.

✓ Your babies' bellies should be against the side of your belly. They shouldn't be turned in any way. Belly-to-belly promotes a good latch.

✓ Don't bend over and bring your nipples to the babies. Instead, bring the babies up to your nipples. Otherwise, your back will break! Use your nursing pillow as support. In fact, in my early days, I used two nursing pillows around me for added height!

2. Rest and Relax

Everyone who has ever had children will tell you to "sleep when the babies sleep." Well, this doesn't work with twins. You have two very different people with two potentially different sleep cycles. (Think about the kicking in the womb...were both babies always awake at the same time? Probably not...) Yes, you should work to finesse the same sleep cycles for your babies, but they will likely want to sleep at different times as newborns. Therefore, please refer to Chapter 3 in regard to creating "day" versus "night." In Chapter 3, I also recommend making "day" begin when you are ready to wake rather than when the sun rises. That way, you can sleep in a bit. This will be your opportunity to catch up on sleep rather than napping during the day. You will more than likely find that when one twin falls asleep, the other wakes up. This can happen all day long, so go to bed early and sleep in!

Another recommendation that I truly had a hard time with was accepting HELP. If you've nursed and one twin falls asleep but the other is cranky and screaming, ask for help from a family member or friend. In my case, my parents drove seven hours to help me for a full week, yet I was allowing myself to become sleep deprived because I felt I had to be "Superwoman" to keep up the housework, cooking, and breastfeeding/baby care. Let those who want to help you do so! You don't have to be "Superwoman." You need a break too! You are no good to the babies if your health is diminished due to lack of rest.

About relaxing, if you are tense, it's hard to get your milk to squirt. I can attest to this personally. Your milk ejection reflex definitely becomes impaired or slowed if you are not in a relaxed state. Therefore, sit in a comfortable position in a comfortable room with a comfortable temperature. I also kept the radio on (See Chapter 3 on creating a nursery environment), which helped me to relax as well. Sometimes I even meditated or prayed while nursing to relax! Just don't think about things you have to do or create mental grocery lists...this will not help.

3. Eat Well to Make Good Quality Milk

DO NOT DIET! I repeat, DO NOT DIET! You need to eat well and eat enough to make good quality and quantities of milk. By breastfeeding twins, I promise you that your weight will return to your normal range very quickly (within three to five months). I was five to seven pounds away from my normal weight through the babies' first year because the body holds onto those extra fat stores in the breasts, thighs, and tummy to support breastfeeding two babies. Once I weaned the babies to cow's milk at a year (which dropped breastfeedings to twice per day), the last five to seven pounds vanished! Trust nature! Don't worry about your sexy jeans that you are yearning to get into...you will, just give it time. In the meantime, go out and treat yourself to a new pair of sexy jeans for now.

Nutrition to Support Breastfeeding Twins
As I have mentioned, you need enough calories to make good quality and quantities of milk. You will also need extra nutrition to support a milk supply for two babies. As a Registered Dietitian, I couldn't believe how much I was eating during my babies' early days of life. I couldn't get enough food! "Good" healthy food and "bad" foods alike: I needed both to support my calorie needs. In addition, I consciously knew that I needed additional fluids based on my nutrition knowledge, but I never could even guess prior to this experience how much water I would truly end up drinking! (See # 4 for fluid recommendations.)

To date, there are no governmental nutrition recommendations for mothers nursing multiples. In my experience, I ate such large quantities of food that I made those around me nauseous. In addition, I never could imagine drinking so much water, but I craved it! I also found myself craving milk and dairy foods constantly and iron-rich foods on occasion. And I believe in the philosophy that if your body needs it, you will crave it! (This pertains to healthy foods rich in vitamins and minerals, not sweets or caffeine! If you crave sweets, go ahead and eat them in moderation...not in excess! And avoid caffeine if you don't want agitated babies!)

I did some digging around...No dietitians I surveyed could point me to any recent research on calorie, fluid, calcium, or iron needs for mothers nursing multiples. I finally scoured the Internet! I should have known to check out the Food and Nutrition Board of the National Academy of Sciences, the creators of the DRIs (Dietary Reference Intakes). Short and sweet: There are no nutritional recommendations to date for mothers breastfeeding more than one baby. The DRI Report from The Food and Nutrition Board (2004), however, does make general recommendations for lactating women to include an increase in fluids while continuing to consume adequate amounts of calcium and iron. Read on for more complete recommendations!

✓ Generally speaking, calorie needs increase about 200-500 per day for mothers nursing one baby. *Therefore, mothers nursing twins need an additional 400-1,000 calories per day.* *

* If you really want to determine how many extra calories you will need, visit: www.nap.edu. Search "Dietary Reference Intakes Energy," click on the book, and read pgs. 4-5, 35, & 195-203.

First of all, heed this advice: Eat when you are hungry and stop when you are full. Eat a varied diet with many nutritious foods including high-fiber whole grains, fruits, and vegetables.

Eat to hunger, and drink to thirst. Your body will tell you how many calories to eat. Just make sure what you are eating is well balanced, and don't waste calories on "junk foods" or sugar-sweetened beverages like soda, juice, iced teas, and other similar beverages. In fact, your best beverage choices are water and nonfat milk. (I'll explain this in the next section.)

Don't feel guilty about consuming what you may think is a large amount of food...you need it to make good quality milk. However, you should **NOT** be gaining weight during this time frame. You should be very slowly *losing* weight. And I don't recommend using a scale to determine if you've lost weight; instead, discover your weight loss by noticing that once-tight clothing now fits or has become loose. The goal for now is not to get into pre-pregnancy clothing; instead, the goal is to provide your twins with the best and most nutritious milk possible!

✓ **Keep this in mind! When breastfeeding, your needs or DRIs (Dietary Reference Intakes) for the following nutrients will increase:**

- Vitamin A, vitamin C, vitamin E, thiamin, riboflavin, niacin, vitamin B_6, folate, vitamin B_{12}, pantothenic acid, biotin, choline, chromium, copper, iodine, manganese, molybdenum, selenium, zinc, potassium, total water (from food and drinks), carbohydrate, fiber, and protein (Food and Nutrition Board, 2004).

What does all this mean? Why do I need to know this?

Basically, keep taking your prenatal vitamin and eat a well balanced diet to meet your increased vitamin and mineral needs. (Read on for specifics.)

✓ Based on the United States Department of Agriculture's (USDA) (2006) "My Pyramid" guidelines for the 3,000 calorie level (an estimate based on 500 extra calories for nursing each baby), to breastfeed twins exclusively, **you may need up to:**

Food Group	# Servings per day	Serving Sizes
Grains	10 oz.	1 oz. each: ½ to 3/4 cup; 1 slice
Vegetables	4 cups	1 cup cooked or fresh; and 2 cups salad greens = 1 cup serving of veggies
Fruits	2 ½ cups	1 cup or 1 fresh; and ½ cup dried fruit = 1 cup serving of fruit
Milk/Dairy	3 + cups	1 cup = 8 oz.: milk, yogurt, cottage cheese, ice cream, pudding made with milk; OR 1.5 oz. (~ 2 slices) or 1/3 cup cheese = 1 cup serving of dairy
Meats& Beans	7 + oz.	3 to 4 oz. meat looks like a deck of cards; 1 oz. = 1 egg; ½ oz. nuts/seeds, 1 T. nut butter; ¼ cup dry beans/meat substitute
Oils/Fats	10 teaspoons	1 teaspoon oil or tub margarine, 1 oz. nuts

Remember, each person has individualized calorie and nutrient needs. This chart is only a guide, not a definitive meal plan. Listen to your own body to meet your calorie needs. All in all, the most important recommendation here is to consume adequate dairy to preserve your bone health.

A Well Balanced Diet for Nursing Twins
Summed up, you should eat more, drink more water, and continue your prenatal vitamin. Listen to your body – eat when hungry and stop when full. And absolutely drink water when thirsty plus more. I also recommend beginning a DHA supplement (docosahexaenoic acid, an omega-3 fatty acid) like Expecta® Lipil® (created by Enfamil®) once daily during the latter part of your pregnancy and throughout your time breastfeeding to promote eye and brain development of your twins (Mead Johnson & Co.®, 2004). (I preferred Expecta® Lipil® to other standard fish oil supplements since the DHA came from a plant in the sea, Crypthecodinium cohnii oil, rather than coming from fish, which has the potential for mercury contamination.) Talk to your OB-GYN and pediatrician about DHA supplements, and ask if they have particular recommendations. Finally, read on for more information about the recommended servings and food groups from the new USDA "My Pyramid."

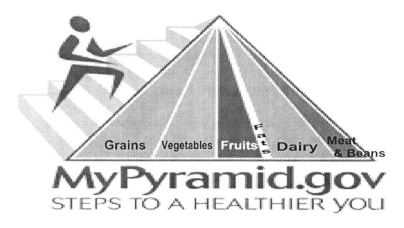

Source: United States Department of Agriculture

✓ **Grains** – Approximately 10 servings daily. The new "My Pyramid" recommends making "half your grains whole." This suggestion means that you should choose at least 5 or more servings of whole grains or high fiber foods. A high fiber food has 3 grams of fiber or more per serving. Check out the nutrition facts label to see how much fiber is in your food choice. You need at least 25 to 35 grams of fiber daily.

✓ **Vegetables** – 4 cups daily. The new pyramid recommends that you "vary your veggies." Each week, you should aim for 3 cups of dark greens, 2 ½ cups orange veggies, 3 ½ cups dry beans and peas, 9 cups starchy veggies, and 10 cups of other veggies. With vegetables, the more the better! Don't restrict yourself...Just be careful with what you're putting ON your veggies. (See "Fats" for more details.) And stick to fresh or frozen vegetables instead of canned veggies, which can be high in sodium!

✓ **Fruits** – Approximately 2 ½ cups daily. The new pyramid recommends eating a variety of fruit and limiting fruit juices.

In my professional opinion, everyone, including children and especially babies, should avoid fruit juice. Here's why: When you drink the juice instead of eating the fruit, you're missing out on healthy fiber. Also, when you eat the fruit, you're eating one piece of fruit. Do you know how many oranges it takes to make a 4 oz. glass of juice (which is the serving size)? A lot more than one! Eat the fruit instead. You can also think of it this way...a 12-ounce soda, which is sugared water, has 41 grams of sugar, or 10 ½ teaspoons. A 12-ounce glass of orange juice, which yes, has vitamin C but very little fiber, has **42 grams** of sugar, or 10 ½ teaspoons! Juice, in my book, is equal to soda in regard to sugar content...pure junk! And if you wouldn't give your infant a sippy cup of soda, then don't give them a sippy cup of juice (which can cause severe diaper rash anyway because of the high acid content in juice)!

✓ **Dairy** – 3 + cups. When I first discovered higher dairy recommendations in my lactation research, I was appalled. I thought, "There's no way!" Then, I added up my daily dairy servings while breastfeeding twins.

Here, I'll show you:

- *Morning* – 24 oz. nonfat milk with my oatmeal (plus 8 oz. nonfat milk used in preparing the oats)
- *Lunch* – 2 pieces of American cheese on my sandwich, 8 oz. low-fat yogurt
- *Dinner* – 1/3 cup cheese sometimes sprinkled on my meal
- *Nighttime snack* – cereal with 16 oz. nonfat milk

For a grand total of = 9 SERVINGS!

(Remember, a serving is 8 oz. milk or yogurt or 2 pieces of cheese.)

I consumed on average nine servings of dairy products daily. I craved dairy, and I listened to my body. But why does a woman nursing twins need so many dairy products? CALCIUM! Your babies get their calcium from your milk; and if your calcium intake is low, their calcium will come from *your* bones. Your bones will, in turn, lose density (or in simple terms, *fall apart*). Drink milk and eat dairy for superior bone health!

You can also obtain calcium from non-dairy sources including fish with bones (salmon or sardines), spinach, beans, and calcium-fortified foods (for example, soft tub margarines – careful with those calcium-fortified juices!). Ask your physician about the latest research on the safety of soy since it may pass into breastmilk. Vitamin D, from foods (fortified milk, egg yolks, fatty fish) and sunlight, is just as important to help you to absorb calcium. If you cannot consume the recommended amount of calcium- and vitamin D-rich foods, then you can add a calcium supplement with vitamin D. Ask your obstetrician at your six-week visit or your pediatrician how much calcium plus vitamin D you should take to support nursing twins. One final tip: take your calcium/vitamin D supplement with a meal, but at a different meal from when you take your prenatal vitamin for the best possible absorption.

Then, the question arises: "Low-fat versions or regular dairy?" Although one year olds should consume whole milk to obtain essential fat in their diets, the philosophy of the American Academy of Pediatrics (AAP) (2007) is that **everyone** over the age of two is advised to consume low-fat dairy to reduce saturated fat intake (reducing the risk of heart disease, diabetes, obesity, etc.). Therefore, all Americans age two and older should get down to low-fat (1%) or nonfat (skim) milk for lower cholesterol and better overall health. That said, I will also endorse lower fat dairy products such as yogurt, cottage cheese, and cream cheese. One can very easily switch to these and barely notice a difference in taste.

Sandwich cheese and hard cheese, on the other hand, does lose some taste quality when the fat is reduced. Pre-pregnancy and post-lactation, I used fat-free cheeses to lower the saturated fat in my diet (See "Fats" for more about saturated fat) for overall health and to decrease my risk of heart disease. However, during my pregnancy, fat-free cheese tasted horrific since my taste buds were in an altered state. And during my breastfeeding/lactating days, I was looking for the extra calories and used regular cheeses. That said, I think it is also important to tell you that I am of normal weight and have excellent cholesterol levels. So, choose your cheese wisely. If you are overweight to start and have questionable cholesterol, opt for the low-fat or fat-free cheeses.

✓ **Meat & Beans** – 7 ounces per day. Includes poultry, fish, beans, eggs, nuts, and red meats: beef, pork, lamb, and veal. USDA (2006) suggests "going lean with protein;" but while breastfeeding, continue to consume a variety of protein foods to meet your iron needs.

Two decks of cards worth of protein (lean meat, fish, skinless/boneless poultry) and some dry beans or an egg are plenty. Again, I believe that if you need extra iron, you will crave iron sources or red meat, which is the best absorbable form of iron. You can also add foods high in vitamin C (citrus, spinach, strawberries, kiwi, tomatoes) to iron sources to absorb the iron better. On most days, however, try to choose healthier meats like white meat, skinless poultry, or fish. Your protein foods should be baked or grilled, not fried, and meat cuts should be from the loin or round portion to keep fat content lower. Ground meats, including ground turkey, should be 90% lean or better. Salmon is the best protein choice for you since it is a natural source of DHA, which helps promote eye and brain development in your babies (Mean Johnson & Co.®,

2004). You should strive to eat salmon at least once a week, and it can be eaten safely up to two times a week while lactating. Don't forget about non-meat sources of protein. Beans, peas, and nuts are wonderful, heart healthy foods that can provide iron as well. Keep in mind that if you consume vitamin C foods along with beans, peas, and nuts, you can absorb the iron more effectively. Just keep in mind that beans may cause you and your babies to become gassy. If this happens, you can limit them and then add them back to your diet when your babies start solids.

✓ **Oils/Fats** – 10 teaspoons daily, but not all fats were created equal...

- *Monounsaturated Fat* – Good fat that can help lower cholesterol; therefore, use this type of fat in moderate amounts daily. Monounsaturated fats come from olive oil, peanut oil, canola oil, nuts, and avocado.

- *Polyunsaturated Fat* – OK fat; again, use this type of fat in moderate amounts. Polyunsaturated fats come from safflower, corn, sunflower, soybean, and other "vegetable" oils. Also, the WONDERFULLY HEALTHY "*omega-3's*" are in this group!

  - *Omega -3 fatty acids* (which have DHA) have numerous health benefits since they have anti-inflammatory properties.

  - Consume *omega-3 fats* regularly from salmon, walnuts, and an occasional egg yolk.

- *Saturated fat* – "Not so good" fat; raises cholesterol and can lead to heart disease. Therefore, limit saturated fat. Comes from animal fats (meat, whole milk, sour cream, cheese, organ meats, egg yolks, poultry skin, and butter) and also palm oil and coconut oil.

- *Trans fat* – The worst fat; raises cholesterol and lowers good cholesterol! Also known as "partially hydrogenated" oils found in some snack foods and most fast foods. No amount is safe! Occurs when liquid vegetable oils are transformed into a solid form at room temperature (for example, stick margarine). Look for trans on the labels and avoid it at all costs!

Remember, fats are also found naturally in many foods and unnaturally in many sweets. Be aware of this when splurging on a dessert or junk food item. Most of your fats should come from the healthy food sources rather than from sweets or junk foods. And avoid fast food altogether! As mentioned, use olive or canola oil in cooking, and only use light tub margarines since these don't have trans fat. Also, choose lower fat or light versions of salad dressings, mayonnaise, ice cream, etc. if you consume these on a regular basis. Remember, all foods can fit in moderation! (NOTE: Diets too low in fat may produce breastmilk with a lower fat content, which can be dangerous to the developing baby. Therefore, avoid being *too restrictive* with fats.)

All in all, eat many different foods in moderation. If you want to splurge on something that isn't so healthy, just be sure you've had well balanced meals throughout the day including calcium-rich dairy foods, fruits, vegetables, and high-fiber whole grains. Finally, if you are noticing that certain foods make you gassy (broccoli, beans, cabbage, onions, etc.), these may also make your baby gassy! If you notice this, make a list of which foods are offenders and avoid them until your babies are four to six months old.

Herbs
Breastfeeding literature commonly makes mention of "milk enhancing" herbs. Be careful what you take, as herbs are not regulated by the Food and Drug Administration (FDA) and may be unsafe. In fact, they may not even contain the herb they are supposed to contain. Ask your physician before taking any herbs, over the counter medications, or prescription medications.

4. Stay Hydrated for Good Quantities of Milk

My first piece of advice is to invest in a water cooler and safe water from a spring. Don't assume that because your water is from your own well that it is safe. And don't assume that if you have a water filter for your city water that it is safe also. Well water can be high in nitrates, which can cause "blue baby syndrome" (See Appendix C). Well water can also be contaminated without you even knowing it. City water can be high in chlorine or other minerals that may not be filtered out with your filtration unit. Go for water from a spring! See Appendix C for more information on safe water.

I went through about 4 - 5, five gallon bottles of water in two weeks! This may seem like a lot, but you become VERY thirsty when breastfeeding twins. And you mustn't let yourself dehydrate (one sign of the beginnings of dehydration is very dark or brownish urine). It is absolutely essential that you drink enough water.

While I could find NO literature on fluid recommendations for mothers nursing twins, I will provide you with a few suggestions based on what I did (since I successfully made lots of milk for over a year!) and based on the suggestions from many reputable breastfeeding organizations:

1. Drink when you are thirsty and drink often throughout the day.

2. Drink as much as it takes to quench your thirst.

3. Get a 30 oz. or larger cup for your water. You will probably be thirsty for a full glass after each feeding. (Remember; quench your thirst...don't make yourself nauseous!)

4. In your babies' early months, keep a pitcher of water full and nearby at all times.

5. At night, have two pitchers of water on your nightstand. After nighttime feedings, fill your glass and drink to quench your thirst before you go back to sleep.

6. At first, you may urinate more often than usual (about as much as that last trimester of pregnancy), but your body will adjust to your increased fluid intake.

7. Your urine should be pale yellow or clear-ish. If your urine is bright yellow or brown, you may be headed towards dehydration.

8. Dehydration may make your milk supply decrease; so don't get to this point!

9. Your only beverages should be water and nonfat milk.

While breastfeeding twins, it's no doubt that you will be very thirsty. Choose water to keep hydrated instead of choosing other beverages. If you choose instead to drink juices, sodas, or any other sweetened beverages, you will have a major problem: WEIGHT GAIN! All those sweetened beverages, *including* 100% juice, have calories (about 150 or more calories in 12 ounces, to be exact). Meeting your high fluid needs by drinking sweetened beverages can then lead to weight problems from all the extra "empty" calories.

Empty calories have no nutrition and therefore no use in the body; and thus become energy stores (FAT STORES!). Drinking only water and nonfat milk can help you avoid those excess empty calories. And if you really want to get into some of those pre-pregnancy clothes soon, definitely avoid sugar sweetened beverages and juices!

I also want to mention diet beverages and caffeine. Today, diet beverages are made with any of the following chemicals or combination of chemicals: aspartame (Equal), saccharin (Sweet and Low), acesumfame K, sucralose (Splenda), or sugar alcohols (end in –ol such as xylitol, malitol, manitol, sorbitol). These are CHEMICALS! We truly don't have enough long-term studies to determine safety during pregnancy or lactation, so my advice is to avoid them. Why put chemicals that may be harmful for your tiny babies into your breastmilk? No need! Drink water or nonfat milk instead. If you need a little sweetness, add some chocolate syrup to your milk. Better safe than sorry!

As for caffeine, it is said by some obstetricians that excessive caffeine can induce miscarriage. In addition, we also know that caffeine is a stimulant and is addictive. Therefore, why drink it and put it into our breastmilk? Would you feed your tiny babies coffee in a bottle? Well, essentially, drinking coffee regularly and frequently will do just that. Don't risk it!

What about alcohol? Many medical authorities have debated the safety of drinking alcohol on occasion while nursing. It does pass into breastmilk, so you will give your baby a "buzz." Many moms decide to stop drinking altogether until after they've stopped breastfeeding, and others come up with strategies like drinking right after a feeding or after the last feeding of the day when the babies are sleeping through the night. My philosophy is to avoid alcohol. Is it really worth putting something that kills brain cells into your breastmilk? Also, it is a MTYH that certain types of alcohol increase breastmilk supply.

Alcohol is absorbed into fat cells and then gets metabolized by the body. Women have more fat stores than men, and it therefore takes longer for alcohol to leave a woman's body than a man's. Therefore, even if you try one of the aforementioned tricks, you still may have some alcohol in your breastmilk. It's only for a year or so that you'll be nursing, and then you can have a drink whenever you want. So I say, give up drinking alcohol for the time being!

What about Exercise? Limit it for Now...
Other health authorities may or may not agree with me on this one, but it is my opinion that exercise can be harmful during the first four months of breastfeeding twins. I'm *not* talking about going for a nice stroll through the mall or neighborhood. Please do this for sanity and the reduction of cabin fever! The exercise I'm referring to makes you sweat, makes your cheeks red, and brings

your heart rate up to where you feel it beating. This type of cardiovascular exercise is normally very healthy, and I encourage you to begin this well into breastfeeding your twins, at about the four-month mark. But extreme exercise while nursing newborn twins may pose some milk supply issues:

1. Extreme exercise can cause mild or even severe dehydration, which may cause your milk supply to dwindle.

2. You already need so much fluid, and exercise causes you to need even MORE fluid. Can you drink enough to make up for your fluid losses? It would take a lot of fluid!

3. Extreme exercise burns a lot of calories...calories which you need for energy and for good quality breastmilk! You'd need to eat even more to compensate!

In my experience, the benefits of exercise did not outweigh the risk of affecting my quality and quantity of milk. I wanted my twins to get as much milk as they needed and the best quality nutritious milk possible. Therefore, I chose not to exercise until my babies were six months old. Yes, I went on leisurely strolls a few times a week (and don't forget about the 700 trips up and down the stairs, the house cleaning, and the laundry room trips), but I didn't go out running for a five-mile jog or to the gym for an hour. Had I had one baby, I probably would renew my gym membership knowing that I could make up for lost fluids and calories. But with two babies for which to provide milk, I decided not to exercise.

But I didn't sit on the couch eating bon-bons either. I want to make it very clear that I do not endorse a sedentary lifestyle. During my early days with the twins, I never once turned on the TV. I kept busy with housework and writing during nap times; and during "awake" time, we played, read books, nursed, laughed, and did other baby things. I NEVER sat on the couch and therefore did not consider myself inactive or sedentary. And as soon as nursing was well established, believe me, I got on the treadmill to work up a good sweat!

Also know that excessive exercise can leave behind some lactic acid in your body from your muscles working hard. Lactic acid can make your milk taste weird for your babies. If you do choose to exercise, drink lots of water to help your body get rid of the lactic acid.

5. Nurse Often, Pump Wisely, and NEVER Use Formula

(If your pediatrician has recommended formula for medical purposes or in cases of failure to thrive, please follow your physician's advice.)

When I say NEVER use formula, I am referring to those people who are feeling concerned because they cannot see an *amount* on a bottle and therefore worry their babies aren't getting enough milk from their breasts. Remember, if your babies are growing steadily and peeing and pooping regularly, they are getting enough milk. Trust the process and trust your body! Breastfeeding is a matter of supply and demand, so if your body needs to make milk for two babies, it will. Trust nature!

I had this fear, but when my twins were growing at the rate of two pounds per month, my fear was quieted. Then, at six months, my twins went from nursing for 20 minutes or more to nursing for 10 minutes or less. In my head, yes, I knew that they were probably becoming more efficient. However, I worried about my milk supply. But sure enough, they gained another one and a half pounds each per month and were peeing and pooping very regularly. I had to keep telling myself that I was doing a fine job with my milk supply.

For those babies with medical issues who need supplemental breastmilk or formula, please listen to your physician. Also, based on the American Academy of Pediatrics, if your babies ever become listless or appear to be dehydrated (less than four wet diapers in a day), please seek medical attention immediately. As for how much pee and poop is enough, please refer to Chapter 8, in the "Diapers" section.

Nurse and pump often and on demand to make the most milk. Essentially, your babies control your milk supply, so let them nurse when they are hungry. In the beginning, they may want to sleep more than nurse and you may have to wake them for feedings. Wake them, try to keep them awake for a 20-minute feeding, and then pump! (See Chapter 11 for more information on pumping.)

In those very early days up until your pediatrician recommends stopping pumping, pump after each feeding to keep your milk supply flowing. I pumped after every feeding until my twins were two months old, which increased my milk supply very well. Then, after two months, my babies' suckling alone was best at keeping my milk supply up.

As the babies continue to grow, they may want to nurse every one and a half to two hours. Let them...they will eventually become more efficient! Remember to follow their lead and not schedules. Also know that as they get older, the time between feedings will increase. By two months old, I was nursing every two hours and pumping after every other feed. By four months, I was still nursing every two hours. But I was no longer pumping because my pediatrician said that I could stop, and I also had a good supply in my deep freezer. By six months, the babies wanted five to six feedings a day and feedings were three to four hours apart, lasting only five minutes each! As time goes on, the breastfeeding multiples experience becomes much easier and very rewarding.

If you have questions regarding when you should pump, how often you should pump, and how long you should continue pumping once your breastmilk supply is well established, talk to your pediatrician. His or her guidelines will be based on your unique life situation and your babies' needs. (General pumping guidelines are in Chapter 11, and more information on storing and handling breastmilk safely is in Appendix B.)

6. Get a Good Support System and Ask Them for Help

When my babies came home from the hospital, I took a "Superwoman" approach and tried to do it all: baby care, housework, cooking, etc. My husband was home from work and my parents and sister were staying with me, but I still felt like I had to do EVERYTHING myself. And then I had a HUGE emotional breakdown...

Let others help you. In fact, ask them to help you! There are people that love you and support your breastfeeding 100%, so delegate tasks for each person in your support system. Ask friends to bring dinner, ask your mom to do some laundry, and have your spouse do the dishes. Have your dad wash the floors, and ask your sister to change a few diapers or help with bath time. All these people would LOVE to help you, and you NEED to let them. Don't burn yourself out. Your sole job for now is breastfeeding your twins! And in the beginning, it's a full-time position with overtime and no time off!

Ask others for help with the babies, cooking, cleaning, etc. and have a friend or family member in mind who will lend a shoulder to cry on or an ear to listen. You need support more than ever in the beginning days, so get your support system lined up before you get home from the hospital. People will love to come over and see the babies, so delegate tasks while they're visiting. I promise, they won't mind!

Going back to what I just said ("people will love to come over"), I must remind you to enforce some boundaries. Ask your friends and family members to call before coming over because you and your babies need to rest. And if you are not up to visitors, it is important that you tell them for your babies' and your own health. Be especially careful if your babies have just come home from the hospital: they may be overly sensitive to commotion and noise, and their immune systems may be immature. The slightest stress can impair their nursing, which can greatly impair their health. If you were never an assertive person, now is the time to change because your babies' health depends on it!

Enforce strict hand washing before others hold the babies, and don't allow children to visit until your pediatrician permits this. Don't allow rude parents to bring their boogery kids over...it may cause one or both of your twins a hospital stay since their immunity may not yet be strong. Don't feel badly putting your foot down. You may hurt others' feelings temporarily, but it's better than subjecting your babies to illness, which could ultimately lead to hospitalization. Use your best judgment; and when needed, say that your doctor does not want other children around the babies until they are "x" weeks or months old.

As I mentioned earlier in this chapter, remember to make friends with your lactation consultant. Contact her as needed and send her thank you cards for all her help. Lactation consultants truly are the ones who teach you HOW to nurse twins, so they are the most vital part of your support system.

Lastly, accept help from those who have breastfed babies. They may have many good tips, and they may be able to empathize with you through the tough times. If some of their advice, however, seems strange, run it by your lactation consultant, physician, or pediatrician. And avoid those formula people who disagree with breastfeeding – they won't help you!

I had one particular family member who thought breastfeeding would hurt my small babies by not providing enough nutrition. She could not see the quantity and assumed that I was underfeeding my babies. If you have one of these in your family, ignore them! She was so wrong; and each time my babies gained two or more pounds in a month from my breastmilk alone, she was the first person I would call with the news!

7. Stay Motivated

Easier said than done...you need to stay motivated. Use positive self-talk constantly. If it is a tough time, tell yourself that it is only temporary and then talk to someone who can help. If it is a breastfeeding problem, call your lactation consultant. If it is an emotional problem, call a friend or family member, or make an appointment with a licensed professional counselor.

If you feel like you've lost possession over your body or that your days are spent ONLY breastfeeding, take the time to rediscover yourself, your talents, and your interests. Pump milk and let your spouse baby-sit while you go out shopping. Or do something you used to love before the babies came along while someone watches the babies. Make some time for you, and take good care of yourself. If you're not in the best physical and mental health, you're no good to your babies.

Some ways I kept motivated to continue breastfeeding:

✓ Watch those babies grow. Take lots of pictures regularly and put them in albums. Every so often, peek at how big they've gotten from YOUR milk!

✓ Think about all the people who said that you couldn't do this...and think about how successful you've been! Call those people and brag about your babies' growth and immunity!

✓ Keep reminding yourself that tough times are only temporary. Think about how much time has gone by since the day the twins were born and how quickly that time flew. You won't have to breastfeed forever.

✓ Think about all the money you are saving by breastfeeding. Go online shopping or to the mall to treat yourself since you've saved your family so much money!

✓ Look at your friends who have babies and aren't breastfeeding...you're almost into all your pre-pregnancy clothing. Are they?

✓ Talk to pregnant women and new moms and share your knowledge. You're truly an expert if you can breastfeed twins!

Chapter 6:
Money Saving Tips for Parents of Twins

1. Breastfeed your twins!

2. Watch for sales in store ads. Compare prices and know the common prices of items you regularly purchase.

3. Clip coupons from the newspaper, but only for items you already use and buy.

4. Have family members and friends clip coupons for you as well, especially for diapers.

5. Switch to store-brand products. In many cases, they work just as well!

6. Ask your favorite baby stores, baby clothing stores, and other stores with a significant baby section if they have a twin discount. For example, OshKosh B'Gosh® offers 10% off every time you shop if you have twins, and Burlington Coat Factory® offers a discount on the second item if you purchase two of the same item for twins.

7. Go to websites of all the products you use and sign up for coupons or e-coupons that you can print from your home computer. For example:

   ✓ www.beechnut.com/
   ✓ www.gerber.com/
   ✓ www.us.pampers.com
   ✓ www.huggiesbabynetwork.com
   ✓ www.luvs.com/en_US
   ✓ www.baby.com (Johnson & Johnson®)

8. Go to your favorite store and grocery store websites and sign up for coupons or free samples of products you use:

   ✓ www.walmart.com
   ✓ www.target.com
   ✓ www.kmart.com

9. At the customer service counter of your grocery stores, sign up to get a savings card. Sometimes grocery stores have baby programs too. Ask about these and sign up! Or visit their websites for more info on such programs or for coupons!

10. Shop on double- or triple-coupon days, or go shopping on "Senior Citizen" day with someone 60+ to get their discount!

11. Sign up for product rewards programs and save points from packages to get money back. Check company websites to see what current promotions are running. For example:

    ✓ Pampers® has offered the "Gifts to Grow" program whereby you save codes from a sticker inside your pack of diapers/wipes and accumulate points. After you have so many points, you can choose certain gifts (toys, books, etc.).

    ✓ Beechnut® has had a program whereby you save proofs of purchase and get money back towards your future baby food purchases.

    ✓ Gerber® runs similar promotions where you save proofs of purchase to get coupons in the mail.

12. Shop at the end of each season for NEXT year...you can get great buys!

13. Cook larger quantities of food and eat or freeze leftovers. This will prevent the need for takeout/restaurant food since it truly ends up costing more (to your wallet AND your waistline!).

14. Do a search for websites that offer free stuff or coupons. Some examples:

    ✓ www.babytalk.com
    ✓ www.walmart.com

15. Some moms use a cheaper brand of diapers when at home and a better brand for nighttime and outings.

16. Have a yard sale to make some money on things you no longer want, and visit yard sales of people you know who have small children!

17. Buy transition clothing for yourself at yard sales...there's nothing like a "new" pair of jeans that only cost a dollar for the post-pregnancy timeframe!

18. Borrow or obtain baby supplies and clothing from friends or relatives. If you borrow cribs or other similar supplies, check the Internet for the most up-to-date safety standards. You can do this by checking the manufacturer's website. If items are deemed unsafe, toss them in the trash! For more on safety ratings and recall information, visit:

   ✓ www.cpsc.gov/
   ✓ www.consumer.gov
   ✓ www.consumerreports.org
   ✓ www.ftc.gov/ftc/consumer/home.html
   ✓ www.thefirstyears.com/
   ✓ www.recalls.gov
   ✓ www.greatestsource.com/Greatest_Source/RECALLS_greatestRECALLS.html

19. Buy and sell on www.ebay.com. Look for inexpensive baby clothing or other baby stuff. Remember to check safety standards and recalls before obtaining any baby products.

20. Love photos? Shop around online to find cheap photo developing sites. This will also save you on time since you can download photos from home and have them shipped to your mailbox. My favorite is www.walmart.com.

21. Go to www.upromise.com, register credit cards and store cards, and start saving for college for your babies!

22. These suggestions may not save you money, but they may help others immensely by saving THEM money:

   ✓ Donate your breastmilk to milk banks for mothers who have premature babies or ill babies. These mothers may need your milk until their milk comes in, or they may be adoptive parents who cannot successfully induce lactation. (See Chapter 7 for more info on the National Milk Bank: www.nationalmilkbank.org/)

   ✓ Donate those "free" cans of premature or regular infant formula to hospitals' neonatal intensive care nurseries.

Chapter 7:
My Favorites

My Favorite Pregnancy/Baby Books

✓ *Your Pregnancy Week by Week,* by Glade B. Curtis and Judith Schuler, Da Capo Press, 2004

✓ *Girlfriends' Guide to Pregnancy,* by Vicki Iovine, Pocket Books, 1999

✓ *When You're Expecting Twins, Triplets, or Quads,* by Barbara Luke and Tamara Eberlein, HarperCollins Publisher Inc., 2004

✓ *What to Expect When You're Expecting,* by Arlene Eisenberg, Heidi Murkoff, and Sandee Hathaway, Workman Publishing, 2003

✓ *What to Expect the First Year,* by Arlene Eisenberg, Heidi Murkoff, and Sandee Hathaway, Workman Publishing, 2002

✓ *Your Baby's First Year,* by Stephen P. Shelov, Bantam Books/American Academy of Pediatrics, 2004

My Favorite Breastfeeding Books

✓ *So That's What They're For,* by Janet Tamaro, Adams Media Corp., 2005

✓ *Mothering Multiples,* by Karen Kerkhoff Gromada, La Leche League International, 1999

My Favorite Baby Books

✓ *Twin to Twin,* by Margaret O'Hair and Thierry Courtin, Margaret K. McElderry, 2003

✓ *Hello Twins,* by Charlotte Voake, Candlewick, 2006

✓ Any *Dr. Seuss* books

✓ Any books by Sandra Boynton (*Barnyard Dance, Belly Button Book, Doggies, But Not The Hippopotamus, The Bedtime Book*, etc…They're all great!)

✓ Any books with large bright pictures (especially of babies!)

✓ Any lift-the-flap books or pop-up books

My Favorite Websites

General Baby Information
✓ www.babycenter.com
✓ www.parenting.com
✓ www.twinsmagazine.com
✓ www.aap.org
✓ www.cdc.gov
✓ www.zerotothree.org

(I hate to list formula websites, but they do have some good baby information:)

✓ www.verybestbaby.com (Nestle)
✓ www.enfamil.com/ (Mead Johnson®)
✓ www.welcomeaddition.com/ (Abbott Laboratories®)

Safety Information and Supplies
✓ www.cpsc.gov
✓ www.getonboardwithsafety.com
✓ www.onestepahead.com
✓ www.safercar.gov
✓ www.usa.safekids.org

Product Websites
✓ www.us.pampers.com
✓ www.beechnut.com
✓ www.gerber.com
✓ www.huggiesbabynetwork.com
✓ www.luvs.com/en_US
✓ www.baby.com (Johnson & Johnson®)

Breastfeeding Information
✓ www.lalecheleague.org **AND** 1-877-4 LA LECHE, the NEW Breastfeeding Helpline available 24 hours per day. (See the website for local La Leche League phone numbers for peer leaders/local group meeting times.)

✓ www.4woman.gov/Breastfeeding/
(The Federal Breastfeeding Helpline – Or you can call: 1-800-994-9662)

✓ www.nurseherenow.com (Empowers women to breastfeed anywhere!)

✓ www.breastfeedingpartners.org (Breastfeeding Partners)

✓ www.nursingmothers.org/ (Nursing Mother's Counsel)

✓ www.aap.org (American Academy of Pediatrics)

✓ www.dona.org (Dona International Doula website)

✓ www.cdc.gov/breastfeeding/index.htm
✓ www.medela.com
✓ www.breastfeeding.com
✓ www.breastfeedingbasics.org
✓ www.webmd.com

✓ The African American Breastfeeding Alliance, Inc. – 1-877-532-8535

Becoming a Lactation Consultant
✓ www.lalecheleague.org
✓ www.ilca.org (International Lactation Consultant Association)
✓ www.iblce.org (International Board of Lactation Consultant Examiners – to take the exam to become a lactation consultant)

Medical and Drug Information
✓ Poison Control – 1-800-222-1222 (Memorize this number!)
✓ www.cdc.gov
✓ www.webmd.com
✓ www.healthfinder.gov
✓ www.aap.org (American Academy of Pediatrics)
✓ www.aafp.org (American Academy of Family Physicians)
✓ www.hmhb.org/index.html (Healthy Mothers, Healthy Babies Coalition)

Nutrition Information
- ✓ www.eatright.org (American Dietetic Association)
- ✓ www.mypyramid.gov (USDA Food Pyramid – Counts calories/nutrients too.)
- ✓ www.sbanutrition.com (Great nutrition information for kids!)
- ✓ www.dietitianapril.com (April Rudat's Nutrition Counseling Private Practice)

My Favorite Magazines (These also have great websites!)

- ✓ *TWINS:*   www.TWINSmagazine.com
- ✓ *Parenting:*   www.parenting.com
- ✓ *American Baby:*   www.americanbaby.com
- ✓ *Baby Talk:*   www.babytalk.com
- ✓ *Parents:*   www.parents.com

Other Interesting Multiples Websites

- ✓ www.intltwins.org/ (The International Twins Association)

- ✓ www.marvelousmultiples.com (Marvelous Multiples)

- ✓ www.nomotc.org (National Organization of Mothers of Twins Clubs, Inc.)

- ✓ www.twinhope.org (Twin Hope, Inc. - The International Center for Twin Diseases)

Becoming a Breastmilk Donor

If you have tons of current milk stored in the freezer or if you are willing to pump breastmilk for others since you have such a good supply, having breastfed twins and all, consider becoming a breastmilk donor to help premature babies who need it most!

- ✓ www.breastfeeding.com
- ✓ www.nationalmilkbank.org/
- ✓ www.4woman.gov/Breastfeeding/index.cfm?page=359

Part 11:

All About Boobs

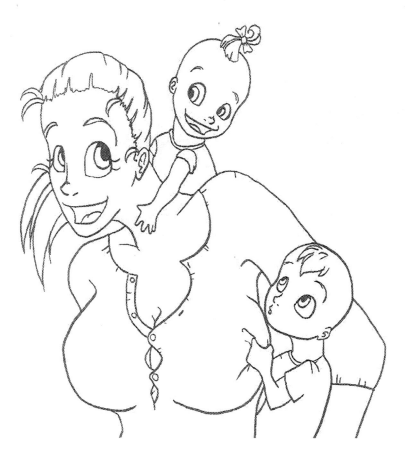

Chapter 8:
Breasts A & P

Breast Anatomy and Physiology – Simple Terms to Know and Understand

There are many different technical terms used when examining anatomy and physiology of female human breasts. In fact, this very natural process is physiologically complex. When completing my research, I couldn't believe what it takes to get milk from the breasts to the babies! I also couldn't believe that after more than 160 years, our knowledge of the anatomy and physiology of the breast has *changed*! I'll explain that more in a bit!

✓ *Breastfeeding/Lactation* – The way nature intended for feeding babies. Although natural, breastfeeding is a learned art requiring much practice.

✓ *Breasts* – While used for fashion purposes and to draw in potential mates pre-pregnancy, these amazing parts of a woman's anatomy serve to feed, nourish, and grow babies both physically and emotionally.

✓ *Nipple* – The sensitive protrusion in the center of the breasts. And nipples are sensitive for a reason: When stimulated, the nerve endings on the nipples make them protrude and become easier for baby to see and suckle (Rosenthal & Arsenault, 2001). Nipples are also moldable so they can form to the unique shapes of babies' mouths (Rosenthal & Arsenault, 2001).

✓ *Areolas* – This darker area surrounding the nipples also secretes milk from many tiny ducts. Like many people, I thought breastmilk was only released from the nipples...not true! Those good old areolas release milk too!

  – Therefore, your babies MUST take your nipples AND your areolas into their mouths to properly latch to get the milk ducts to empty correctly.

✓ *Milk ducts* – Inside the nipple/areola, there are many openings or ducts which transport milk. These ducts branch close to the nipple, and glandular tissue is also found close to the nipple (Ramsay, Kent, Hartmann, & Hartmann, 2005).

- *What does all this mean?* Simply speaking, your babies need to latch properly, taking in the nipple **and** areola, to enable the ducts and glandular tissue to work correctly to release milk.

- Also, your pump attachments need to fit properly around the nipple and areola to stimulate the ducts/glandular tissue, which are found close to the base of the nipple (Ramsay et al., 2005).

- The babies' suckling then triggers the hormone oxytocin, which gets the milk released from your milk ducts out of your nipple and into the babies' mouths.

- The babies also need to breastfeed long enough since breastmilk increases in fat content as a feeding progresses (Ramsay et al., 2005).

✓ *Milk ejection reflex* – Also known as the milk let down reflex. The let down is triggered when the babies begin to suckle the nipple/areola, which causes the subsequent release of the hormone oxytocin. Oxytocin causes the contraction and then ejection of milk from the milk ducts (Rosenthal & Arsenault, 2001).

- You can sometimes feel yourself let down, as it produces a strong, tingly, pins and needles feeling inside your breasts. And when you let down, you can sometimes feel this strong release, and you can hear your babies swallowing like crazy!

- Don't get worried if you don't feel a let down...you may have had one that wasn't as strong. Most women only feel the first let down, which is the strongest. Also know that you let down many times in a breastfeeding session. Don't worry about not feeling a let down...this can stress you, which can delay let down or make it difficult to release your milk.

- In the beginning, let down can occur at any time, which causes leaking. For me, it always happened in the shower in my beginning days of breastfeeding (I started taking my showers AFTER breastfeeding or pumping).

- You can shut off a let down by simply pushing in on your nipples with your forearms GENTLY for a moment (which I did as a teenager at the beach to prevent the cute guys from seeing my erect nipples through my swimsuit after swimming!).

- In the beginning, it can take five to 15 minutes to let down; but as you become more experienced, it may only take one to two minutes to let down (Rosenthal & Arsenault, 2001).

- Lastly, I have to tell you that some women do let down when hearing the cries of another baby, but this NEVER happened to me. In my beginning breastfeeding days, other than letting down while nursing, I let down in the shower, close to the time when the babies typically breastfed, and sometimes when I got cold. Other babies' cries never bothered me. Know that this phenomenon doesn't occur for every breastfeeding mom.

✓ *Oxytocin* – As mentioned, suckling the nipple and areola stimulates the release of this hormone from the pituitary gland, which is responsible for your milk ejection or let down (Rosenthal & Arsenault, 2001). And NEWSFLASH: You will continue to have contractions after giving birth while you breastfeed...this is only temporary. Oxytocin is responsible for triggering these postpartum uterine contractions, which are almost as painful as labor, but these contractions help shrink your uterus back down to its normal, pre-pregnancy size (Rosenthal & Arsenault, 2001).

✓ *Prolactin* – The pattern of pressure and release of the babies' mouths on the areola stimulates the release of prolactin, which is the hormone from the pituitary gland that tells cells to make milk (Rosenthal & Arsenault, 2001). Basically, the more the babies suckle, the more prolactin tells your cells to make milk. This is also known as the supply and demand principle! To keep prolactin levels up, you need nipple stimulation and you need to keep emptying your breasts (Rosenthal & Arsenault, 2001).

✓ *Supply and demand* – Since babies need to suckle for prolactin to be released and signal for the production of more milk, we say that breastfeeding works on supply and demand. Therefore, if two babies are suckling and double the prolactin is being released, there is a signal telling the body to produce double the milk. The more milk that is demanded, the more the body will make for its supply!

✓ *Latching on* – This is the term that describes the correct way for the babies to breastfeed. A good latch includes the babies taking in your nipple AND areola, being in the nose to nipple position, and being in the belly-to-belly position. Also, when the babies are latched properly, you should not hear clicking or smacking sounds.

✓ *Colostrum* – The first amazing secretion from the mammary glands, which usually exists until day two or three after birth, then breastmilk comes in.

  – Colostrum is also known as "liquid gold" since it is yellow-ish and contains powerful and complex antibodies that ward off infection until an infant's own immune system develops further (Rosenthal & Arsenault, 2001).

  – Colostrum is higher in protein and lower in fat than breastmilk, and it is produced in small quantities (Rosenthal & Arsenault, 2001).

  – Colostrum also helps to activate the bowels, which helps the babies pass their first tarry poop called meconium (Rosenthal & Arsenault, 2001).

  – If your babies are premature, you should allow your babies to breastfeed or receive pumped colostrum for its wonderful benefits, but your babies may also need supplemental formula/donor breastmilk until your breastmilk comes in for the additional calories to support optimal growth.

  – If this happens, you must PUMP, PUMP, PUMP to get your milk in so your babies can stop getting formula.

The New Research on Breast Anatomy

Recent research conducted by Ramsay, Kent, Hartmann, and Hartmann (2005) using ultrasound imaging on lactating breasts has shown quite significant changes in breast anatomy. First, Ramsay and others (2005) determined that there are no lactiferous sinuses (pouches that were once thought to contain stored breastmilk). Instead, the authors suggest that milk ducts *transport* breastmilk rather than storing it (Ramsay et al., 2005). Therefore, breastmilk travels through the ducts rather than collecting in areas for storage. It is important to note, however, that breastmilk increases in fat content as breastmilk drains during the breastfeeding session. Therefore, it is important to nurse long enough! Second, Ramsay and others (2005) found that breastmilk ducts branch closer to the nipple and glandular tissue is closer to the nipple. All of this information is very important since babies (or pumps!) must latch properly (taking in the nipple *and* areola) and feed long enough to obtain optimal nutrition.

A Good Latch

Work with your lactation consultant to get both babies to latch correctly. This is something I can explain in words, but it is better to physically work with a lactation consultant to make sure you are doing it right. Some pointers:

✓ Get a good nursing pillow, two nursing pillows, or a twin-specific nursing pillow. Discover which works best for you.

✓ Then, get each baby to master latching on individually.

✓ A good latch includes being belly-to-belly and nose to nipple with a big open mouth that takes in both the nipple and the areola (See photos, next page) (Rosenthal & Arsenault, 2001).

✓ You shouldn't hear any clicking or smacking sounds from the babies. If you do, unlatch the baby with your pinky to break the seal, and then re-latch the baby.

✓ While you are still in the hospital, once both babies get the hang of latching individually, have your great lactation consultant get them both on both breasts at the same time to tandem breastfeed. Do this ASAP! I first tried tandem breastfeeding on day two. Remember, practice makes perfect, and the sooner you can get comfortable with this, the better, since you will have to leave the hospital someday!

✓ Learn to tandem nurse with the help of another person.

✓ Then, when successful at tandem nursing, learn to tandem nurse while alone. (See my "breastfeeding alone" recommendations in Chapter 3, "Creating a Nursery Environment Conducive to Breastfeeding Twins.")

PHOTOS OF A GOOD LATCH

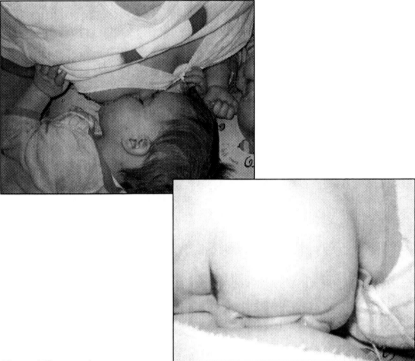

Manual Expression

How to manually express breastmilk in two simple steps:

1. Wash your hands. Place your thumb and pointer finger one inch above and one inch below your nipple.

2. Push in slightly, and then gently squeeze your fingers back towards your nipple (but not on the nipple – no need to squeeze the actual nipple).

For modesty purposes, I will not provide photos of how to manually express milk. Instead, ask your great lactation consultant to *show you* this technique while still at the hospital. It really is quite simple and is NOT painful, as I thought it would be! (Don't try this before you deliver, as nipple stimulation may induce contractions!)

Be Kind To Your Breasts and Nipples

✓ No underwire bras EVER!

✓ Always wear a comfortable bra, even at bedtime (those sports bras that button down the front are great)!

✓ Use plenty of Lansinoh® lanolin cream in the beginning days.

✓ Squirt breastmilk on your nipples regularly.

✓ Always allow your nipples to air dry.

✓ Don't wash your nipples; just let the water in the shower gently hit them. Soap will run onto them, and that is okay. But don't directly apply soap or scrub your nipples.

✓ Sleep on your back as much as possible. Prolonged side or stomach sleeping can compress your milk ducts, resulting in breast problems (Rosenthal & Arsenault, 2001).

✓ Break the breastfeeding seal or latch if you need to re-position a baby rather than pulling him off, which can be quite painful.

  – You can break the seal by putting your pinky finger into baby's mouth and "unlatching" her.

What Have You Heard?

✓ *Have you been told that you "won't be able to make milk" because you have small breasts?* This is NOT true...Take it from a "Nearly A" cup herself! I had PLENTY of milk regardless of my flat-chestedness. In fact, as long as *some* breast tissue exists, breast size has no effect on milk production or quality (Rosenthal & Arsenault, 2001).

✓ *How about large breasts...do you think you might "smother" the babies?* There are positions and pillows available for women with large breasts, which make breastfeeding twins easier. Talk to your great lactation consultant for suggestions!

✓ *Have you heard that you need to "prepare" your breasts by doing "exercises" or by "roughing up" your nipples?* AAP (2004) says there is no need for this, and these techniques can actually lead to preterm labor since nipple stimulation can cause uterine contractions.

✓ *Do you think your nipples are inverted?* Ask your doctor to be sure while still pregnant. People with very inverted nipples can benefit from talking with a lactation consultant prior to delivery.

✓ *Have you heard women talking about "not being able to make milk medically?"* Well, this is extremely rare. Women who cannot make milk medically do not have any glandular tissue at all, but they can take drugs called lactogogues (which stimulate prolactin levels) to attempt milk production. More commonly, women who say they "cannot make milk" more than likely have babies who latch poorly or incorrectly, both of which can be "cured" by a great lactation consultant (Rosenthal & Arsenault, 2001). Or, women may be imposing a timed feeding schedule on their babies or may be supplementing with formula, which both reduce milk supply.

✓ *Have you heard about babies that self-weaned at three months old?* This is typically not "self-weaning." It may be a nursing strike, and there are ways to prevent these (see Chapter 10). Or in some cases when the babies are given bottles, they may develop a preference for the bottle and begin to refuse the breast (also called nipple confusion, see Chapter 10).

✓ *What have you heard about when you should first breastfeed?* AAP (2004) recommends beginning breastfeeding as soon after birth as possible and keeping the babies as close to you as medically possible. After your babies are born, express your wishes for your babies to "room in" with you, if medically possible.

✓ *Should you feed on a schedule?* AAP (2004) says **NO!** You should **feed on demand and as often as necessary** for best success. Some babies, especially preterm babies, may need to be reminded to eat and may need to be awakened for feedings in the early days of life. Your pediatrician can instruct you on this (usually waking them every three or four hours is recommended if they are not waking up themselves for feeds). Remember: crying is a late sign of hunger: so look for *rooting, mouthing, grasping, salivating, hand-to-mouth activity, and/or grimacing* and then BREASTFEED!

✓ *What about c-section recovery?* If you had a c-section, AAP (2004) recommends that you breastfeed as soon as possible after delivery in a semirecumbent position on your hospital bed utilizing pillows on the abdomen.

✓ *How many feedings will newborns need per day?* For newborns, AAP (2004) recommends eight to twelve feedings (or more!) per day, and no more than four hours should pass between night feedings to provide adequate nutrition and hydration for the newborns.

✓ *How to keep track?* Use Feeding Logs! (See Chapter 4.)

✓ *How do you know if the babies are getting enough nutrition/hydration?* AAP (2004) recommends counting the number of wet/dirty diapers per day and monitoring growth. See the guide based on AAP (2004) recommendations, below:

A Quick and "Dirty" Guide on Diapers!

- First 24 hours: At least 1 pee and 1 poopy diaper that will be meconium (thick, black, tarry poop)

- By day three: 3-4 wet diapers and 1-2 stools that are yellowish and no longer meconium

- Later in the first week: 6 wet diapers per day that are pale yellow and a yellow stool with each feeding

- Later in the month: Less stools to include about 3 per day and 6 wet diapers

- After this: Less poop to potentially include a few days going by without any stooling and at least 6 wet diapers (More on this in Chapter 17 in the Diapers section.)

✓ *What about growth...my babies look like they're at the bottom of the growth curves?* AAP (2004) states that the Centers for Disease Control and Prevention (CDC) growth charts are based primarily on infants fed formula (formula-fed babies are typically heavier babies). Therefore, these charts do not "reflect optimal growth associated with breastfeeding" (AAP, 2004). Instead, consider the following:

–   What is most important is that infants should be trending *upward* and not falling on the curve.

- In addition, in April 2006, the World Health Organization (WHO) released new growth charts based on *breastfed* babies internationally. You can download and print these charts, and bring them to your pediatric office to be used in place of the CDC charts.

- Just visit: http://www.who.int/childgrowth/standards/en/ to download these new "Child Growth Standards" charts. Print the "**percentiles**" pages, and ask your nurse to obtain weights and heights in kg and cm since these are not in English measuring units.

✓ *Can I breastfeed if I have diabetes and take insulin?* Yes. You may need to work with your doctor and a registered dietitian to get your blood sugars under good control, but you can breastfeed your babies if you have diabetes and take insulin. You also may need special instructions on how to care for your babies if they have hypoglycemia (low blood sugar) at birth.

Breastmilk for Preterm Babies

According to the AAP (2004), human breastmilk is the feeding of choice, especially for preterm infants. Whether via a feeding tube or other feeding device or from the breast itself, AAP reports that the human milk of mothers who have delivered preterm babies is higher in calories, fat, and protein compared to milk from mothers of term infants (2004). It should be noted, however, that human milk fortifiers or premature infant formula powder (like Similac® NeoSure® Advance® by Abbott Laboratories® or Enfamil® EnfaCare® LIPIL® by Mead Johnson®) are typically added to breastmilk for preterm babies in the beginning weeks of breastfeeding to provide optimal nutrient, vitamin, and mineral intake for optimal growth (AAP, 2004).

Kangaroo Care

Kangaroo care or kangaroo mother care (or kangaroo mother intervention) is, in simple terms, holding your nude (diapered) babies against your bare chest, upright, as constantly as medically possible for skin-to-skin contact, for temperature regulation, and for frequent breastfeeding. Much research has been done on kangaroo care, and the results have shown it to be beneficial and positive, especially for preterm babies. Results of the studies have shown that kangaroo mother care leads to a "bonding effect" between mother and baby, increased feelings of competency for the mother, less nosocomial or hospital-spread infections, and decreased hospital stays (Tessier et al., 1998; Charpak et al., 1997). Fathers can also provide babies with a modified form of kangaroo care by placing them on their bare chests for temperature regulation.

The Breast Crawl
Being with your babies and rooming in, or having your babies constantly in the room with you when medically able, is so important. In fact, this is the first way to succeed in the early days of breastfeeding. You need to see your babies, follow their cues, and breastfeed on demand for best success! Nature intended for you to be close to your babies so that they could suckle as they need to.

The breast crawl is such a cool phenomenon that validates the fact that nature intended for babies to breastfeed and to be close to mom immediately after birth and for the entire hospital stay (if medically possible). What is the breast crawl? Immediately after natural births, when left on mom's tummy, newborns have an inborn and natural ability to *crawl up to the breast*, find the nipple, and initiate suckling (Klaus, 1998). This amazing phenomenon not only serves to provide the newborn with early nutrition and colostrum, but it also serves to provide mother-infant temperature regulation (Klaus, 1998).

Breastmilk's Nutritional Facts

Here are a few interesting tidbits about breastmilk's nutritional properties according to AAP (2004):

✓ The nutrient composition of breastmilk can change through lactation, over the course of a day, within a feeding, or among women!

✓ Women who have preterm babies have breastmilk that is higher in calories, protein, and fat when compared to the milk of women who have term babies...isn't the body amazing?

✓ Breastmilk has a different nutritional breakdown than cow's milk in that breastmilk promotes more rapid gastric emptying and has an immune enhancing effect on the gastrointestinal tract.

✓ In both third world and developed countries, breastfed babies have less gastrointestinal and respiratory diseases and less ear infections when compared to formula-fed babies.

Who Shouldn't Breastfeed

According to AAP (2004), breastfeeding is not recommended in the following situations:

✗ When babies have galactosemia (where the infants cannot have lactose, which is found in breastmilk).

✗ When babies have phenylketonuria, they can only have limited and monitored amounts of breastmilk.

✗ When the mother (in the U.S.) has HIV or human T-cell lymphotropic virus. (Globally, this may be a different situation since the health benefits of breastmilk may outweigh the risk of acquiring HIV.)

✗ When the mother has herpetic lesions to the breast.

✗ When the mother has breast cancer and needs antimetabolite chemotherapy.

✗ If the mother has untreated, active tuberculosis.

✗ When the mother abuses drugs. She can, however, safely breastfeed when off the drugs.

*Before taking ANY drug, be sure to ask your doctor if it is safe while breastfeeding!

Drugs and Breastmilk Interactions

Ask your physician or pediatrician which drugs are safe while breastfeeding. If you think you are in dire need of a particular drug (for example, anti-diarrheals for diarrhea), ask a doctor FIRST before taking it! It can pass into your breastmilk and be harmful to your babies (*Anti-diarrheals for diarrhea should **not** be taken while breastfeeding). If you find lists of breastfeeding-safe medications on the Internet, share these with your doctor and get approval before taking anything first!

In addition, if you accidentally take a drug without even thinking about it, immediately call your babies' pediatrician to see what action to take. Sometimes, the pediatric office may recommend that your babies receive stored, pumped milk in a bottle and that you pump off your milk and toss it for a few hours to protect your babies. But BE SURE to pump at normal feeding times to keep your milk supply up even though you will only be tossing your milk.

Birth Control
Please note that beginning estrogen-containing birth control methods is often a culprit in decreasing milk supply dramatically. If in the past, you typically relied upon birth control to control painful periods, know that by providing breastmilk for two babies, menstruation may be delayed for quite a while. I never got a period until well after my babies' first birthday. If you wish to have birth control methods in place to prevent another pregnancy, talk to your doctor about other options such as condoms or IUDs.

Free Formula

Many other breastfeeding authors make this point, and I feel just as obliged to let you in on a little secret: Formula companies give you free cases of formula, diaper bags, bottle coolers, coupon packs, etc. so that you will use their product, get hooked on it, and *need* to buy it for a whole year for two babies. And mothers of new multiples are a great catch for formula companies! Double the purchases of the stuff! Beware! The nurses aren't just being nice or helpful in giving you free formula or gifts...the formula companies want you hooked so they can get your money for a whole year!

I will be honest: I took the free cases of formula home as a safety net. And you can do the same too. But know that you CAN breastfeed your twins. You DO NOT need formula. And if you make it beyond the nine-month mark, it's pretty safe to say that you won't need that formula after all. Instead, donate the free cases to a local NICU like I did. (See Chapter 23.)

Physiological Jaundice

In simple terms, jaundice is the yellowing of the skin caused by an increase in a substance from the liver called bilirubin, and breastfeeding and pooping will help the jaundiced baby to become less yellow (Rosenthal & Arsenault, 2001). In fact, breastfeeding as long as possible and as often as possible is the best treatment (Rosenthal & Arsenault, 2001). In severe circumstances, phototherapy can be used whereby the baby is put under a bili-light, which looks like a tanning bed for babies. Physicians may also recommend placing the baby in a sunlit window for the same effect to help the bilirubin break down through the skin.

Note: There are other causes of jaundice that should be ruled out by the pediatrician.

"Breastmilk" and "Breastfeeding" Jaundice – Unfair Terminology!

Although I did not experience this, a friend of mine shared her experience of "breastfeeding" jaundice with me. I did not know much about it, so I researched "breastmilk" and "breastfeeding" jaundice so that you, the reader, would have information about this at hand.

What is it?
"Breastmilk" jaundice is really called physiologic jaundice (yellowing of the skin) of newborns, and it is a normal physiologic response to the ingestion of breastmilk (AAP, 2004). "Breastfeeding jaundice," on the other hand, results when the baby or babies are inadequately nursing which then causes increased intensity of the jaundice (AAP, 2004). It can be caused by the babies not suckling well or enough, or it can be caused by mom not making enough milk (because of a poor latch or giving bottles of formula).

The most common treatment for mom and babies is correcting latch problems and *more frequent breastfeeding* to increase babies' intakes and mom's milk supply (AAP, 2004). Pumping after all feedings is also recommended to keep milk supply up. The pediatrician may also recommend that the pumped milk be given to the babies to increase their intake. In advanced cases, pediatricians may recommend phototherapy (putting the babies into what looks like a tanning bed), or they may need to rule out other causes.

Do I need to stop nursing if one or both babies become jaundiced?
No. But, in severe and extreme cases, pediatricians may recommend using formula for one or two days to bring bilirubin levels down (bilirubin causes the yellowing). If your pediatrician insists on this course of treatment, while using the formula, you NEED to pump every time you would have breastfed in order to keep your milk supply up. Also, use orthodontic nipple bottles to prevent nipple confusion. AAP (2004) states that this treatment should be recommended for one to two days, and that a slight recurrence of jaundice when resuming breastfeeding is normal.

Weaning

First of all, when a baby appears to self-wean before nine months old, it is doubtful that he is really self-weaning. If your baby appears disinterested before this time, it is probably a nursing strike. On the other hand, you may wish to wean for personal reasons, at your babies' first birthday, to return to work, or your babies may be getting older and less interested in breastfeeding.

Here are some gentle weaning recommendations:

✓ First and foremost, since the touch and bond of breastfeeding end when you wean, give your children plenty of attention, love, and encouragement for weaning to be a success...Lots of cuddling, snuggling, hugs, and kisses!

✓ Remain child-centered. You can do this by allowing the babies to tell you when they want to wean. Or if you wish to wean sooner than your babies do, you can stop offering a breastfeeding, without refusing breastfeedings altogether.

✓ Don't succumb to pressure by others to wean. Pay no attention to ignorant comments. Wean when you are ready...your breastmilk is still healthy for your babies after one year old, even if you only breastfeed once or twice a day.

I remember my mom telling me that my 21-month old babies were "getting too big" to breastfeed, but I kept going since they were still interested and since I knew the health benefits of breastmilk still exist after the first year!

✓ If you need to wean for a medical emergency, you will have no choice but to wean quickly. Talk to your lactation consultant or OB-GYN for guidelines on weaning for a medical emergency. Otherwise, weaning should be a slow and gradual process for your babies' and your own comfort.

✓ Also, try to avoid weaning in times of transition such as during a move, while on vacation, around the time of a death in the family, etc. Wait until things are pretty settled.

✓ If you wish to wean before your babies turn one year old, you will need to wean your babies to cups or bottles of formula or stored breastmilk. After one year old, wean to *cups* of whole milk or formula. It's a good idea to get your babies used to their next feeding device prior to weaning. It also helps when someone else gives the bottle or cup other than you.

✓ At the time you want to wean, choose the least important feeding to drop first. Be sure to wait a few days before dropping another feeding to be kind to your body (to avoid engorgement and potentially mastitis) and loving to your babies.

✓ For toddlers, when you get down to two feedings (usually morning and night feedings), determine which feeding is least important to them. (This may be the shorter breastfeeding session or the one where they seem more preoccupied.) Or, if your kids can verbalize their wishes, let them decide which feeding they want to end first. Then, work slowly on the last one.

✓ If you become severely depressed and lose interest in things that were once important to you after weaning your babies or at any time postpartum, seek medical attention immediately.

Chapter 9:
Thrush & Plugged Ducts & Mastitis Oh My! (And More!)

First and foremost, I need to share a secret with you. I've already told you to get some good lanolin cream such as Lansinoh®, but here's another secret for nipple success: Get into the habit of regularly squirting breastmilk on your nipples! This may sound weird and perhaps gross (and maybe a little sticky), but it works! For nipple pain and especially for cracked nipples, breastmilk literally works like medicine to help alleviate some of your discomfort. Don't ask me why exactly, but I can attest that it does work based on my experiences!

A Recap of Nipple and Breast Care Tips:

✓ Let your nipples air dry as often as possible.
✓ Don't apply soap (or any other cleansers) directly to your nipples.
✓ Lanolin, Lanolin, Lanolin...after every feeding and pumping (Use those breast pads or you'll have to deal with yellow stains on EVERY bra).
✓ Squirt your milk onto your nipples regularly and let dry.
✓ No underwire bras! But always wear a supportive, *non-underwire*, cotton bra 24 hours a day, seven days a week!
✓ Sleep on your back. Side or stomach sleeping can compress your milk ducts, resulting in breast problems (Rosenthal & Arsenault, 2001).

Read on about some of the pains that can result when you are a breastfeeding mom. And just for your information, I've experienced most of these. Hopefully I can help you not to. Or if you do get any of this stuff, hopefully I can help you get through it with as little pain and as much awareness as possible! A final note: Breastfeeding is so rewarding and amazing that any of these "pains" become insignificant and easily forgettable!

First and Foremost: Sore Nipples

Sad but true...every beginning breastfeeder gets sore nipples. And this is normal since your nipples have never before performed such a task. However, when breastfeeding babies with a good latch, nipple soreness will subside in the first few days when your nipples become "broken in" for their new task at hand.

AAP (2004) states that persistent sore nipples beyond the first four to seven days of lactation often indicate a poor latch. Therefore, if you are experiencing persistent nipple pain, immediately call your lactation consultant to correct a poor latch. Lactation consultants have great tips for correcting such problems. Call your great lactation consultant, the hospital's lactation consultant help line, or refer to Chapter 7 for the La Leche League or the Federal Breastfeeding Helpline's contact information.

Cracked Nipples and Thrush

My babies latched well from the first feeding, so I never truly experienced cracked nipples until I got thrush. You can also prevent cracking by regularly using Lansinoh® cream after every feeding and pumping session in those beginning days. If you are still cracking and think one or both babies are latching improperly, please call your lactation consultant and/or pediatrician.

When my babies were three months old, we decided to throw a Christening party (which was well after their actual Baptism). We felt that this was a safe time to allow a zillion people, including small children, to meet the babies since they had passed the six-pound mark and were deemed healthy enough to be around people by our pediatricians. It was August, and we traveled nine hours by car to get to our hometown for this party. It was hot, and I remember feeling sweaty. My nipples began to itch and burn, and I remember thinking that something seemed wrong with my breasts. I unlatched my nursing bra to let my nipples "breathe," and I hoped this strange sensation would resolve.

I've never been good at solving mysteries. I knew in the back of my mind that Julia had some white spots on her tongue one-week prior, but I never put two and two together. None of my breastfeeding resources mentioned itchy nipples, so I kept nursing through the itchiness. But the itchiness didn't resolve, and my nipples cracked terribly. I swore I would have to quit breastfeeding because the pain began shooting through my breasts. I thought I would die.

I had now begun to suspect that thrush or a fungal yeast infection was the culprit. But none of my breastfeeding books seemed to mention pain associated with thrush. Could this be the culprit? I immediately got both babies to the pediatrician, and sure enough, they both had a terrible case of thrush. Our doctor prescribed one bottle of Nystatin for all three of us to use (which is wrong – you aren't supposed to share prescriptions with anyone!), and none of us were treated properly. My itchiness turned into severe pain, shooting from my nipples inward, and I used a whole container of Lansinoh® to get my cracked nipples to heal. (NOTE: Pat your nipples with a warm washcloth to cleanse them before applying lanolin or medicated creams.)

Since none of us got better, I requested that we all get our own prescriptions (My prescription came from my OB-GYN). It took a good week after receiving the new prescriptions to improve, and then my nipples finally healed. (I also "sterilized" anything that went into the babies' mouths.) The moral of the story and take-home message in this "Cracked Nipples and Thrush" section: Tell your doctor when your babies have white spots *anywhere* in their mouths and get prescriptions promptly for each involved party to prevent this from happening to you. It is not fun. In fact, after having experienced many breast ailments, thrush was by far the most painful (worse than mastitis!).

Common Symptoms of Thrush:
✓ Itchy and/or cracked nipples
✓ Flaky or shiny looking nipples
✓ Nipples that may look discolored or red
✓ Pain that shoots from your nipple inward
✓ Breastfeeding that is so uncomfortable that you think about quitting…Don't! Seek treatment and give yourself time to heal. This is only temporary!

Do continue breastfeeding, and keep in mind that the yeast needs to be killed! Both you and the babies need to use your prescriptions faithfully. Also boil pacifiers, disinfect toys, and wash hands, towels, bras, and clothes frequently. Also, if you use pumped milk, serve it the same day or throw it away. Do not freeze this milk, and boil pump parts to kill the "fungus among us!"

Engorgement

Engorgement is when your breasts are so full of milk that they feel and look like they are going to explode. This occurs when your milk first comes in during your babies' first few days of life, and it can occur again many times throughout your breastfeeding career. In your early breastfeeding days and at other times when you experience engorgement, know that engorgement is temporary and that feeding early, correctly, and frequently is the cure (Rosenthal & Arsenault, 2001). Let your babies (and/or breast pump) do their best to remove the milk!

With twins, specifically, you are making twice the amount of milk; therefore, any change in your breastfeeding routine can lead to engorgement. In addition, whenever a breastfeeding session is missed or when breastfeedings are reduced (due to adding solids or your babies sleeping through the night/taking longer naps), engorgement is likely.

My main cause of engorgement, beyond my initial engorgement when my milk came in, began when my babies started sleeping through the night, thus going longer periods of time between feedings. I re-experienced some engorgement when adding solids as well (since the babies replaced some of their calories with solid food and thus suckled less from the breast). Engorgement can cause your breasts to feel painfully full, and you may feel a burning sensation. Your first instinct may be to pump off the milk to release the discomfort of being so full of milk. In the beginning days of breastfeeding, this is an acceptable approach. However, when your babies are suckling less for a reason (e.g., sleeping through the night or getting extra calories from eating solid foods), pumping off the extra milk is counterproductive since pumping would essentially tell your body to continue making milk as usual.

In the case of your babies sleeping through the night or eating more solid foods, get through a few days of pain. And with each subsequent day, the pain (and amount of milk) will lessen as your body adjusts to what the babies need. If, however, the pain is so severe that you could cry, go ahead and pump for five minutes to relieve the pressure. But don't let it become a habit. Let your body adjust to your babies' changing needs. To alleviate some of the pain, you can try massaging your breasts while in the shower to release some excess milk.

Engorgement essentially causes milk supply to lessen as your babies grow older and need less breastmilk. Your body then adjusts to your babies' changing needs. If, however, you are a new breastfeeding mother and you become engorged from a missed breastfeeding session or another occurrence and you DO NOT want a change or decrease in your breastmilk supply, you must pump off 15 minutes of breastmilk in order to keep your supply up. If your babies are sick and not breastfeeding as long during sessions or as often throughout the day, you need to pump as if you were breastfeeding as usual to keep up your milk supply (Rosenthal & Arsenault, 2001). You can ask your pediatrician how often you should pump based on your babies' age and situation.

You may also experience engorgement if you have plugged ducts. If you have a plugged duct, your milk cannot be released: engorgement. Read on!

Plugged Ducts

Plugged ducts are no fun! Because of a change in your babies suckling, milk may not be released from any given milk duct, causing it to become blocked or plugged. Also, you may feel the need to be sexy and purchase one of those nursing bras with underwires. This will cause plugged ducts! Or you may bump into a wall or run into something, causing a blow to your breast, which can also cause plugged ducts.

To the touch, you may feel a lump on your breast. When you push on the lump, it feels kind of gristly (yes, like gristle on meat). Your nipple may also have a whitish looking "pimple" on it, which is essentially clogged, dried up milk on the surface of your nipple.

To get your duct to unplug, breastfeed, breastfeed, breastfeed! And then get to the shower and make it nice and steamy. Get on in and hit your "lump" or plugged duct with hot water, without scalding yourself, of course! As you let the water hit your breast, massage the lump in circular motions as well from the farthest away part of your breast in towards the nipple to help release the clogged milk. As for the "pimple:" don't try to pop it. Let your babies suckle regularly and vigorously to release the milk and pop this "pimple." In my case, the duct was unplugged before the "pimple" went away. It actually took a month for my nipple to look normal again.

You can also purchase donut-shaped, gel-filled pads in stores that sell breastfeeding supplies. You can wet these and then microwave them (or freeze them and use these for engorgement), and you can then apply these to your breast to help break up the plug. Or, you can wet a washcloth and microwave it in the same way to apply moist heat to the lumpy area. If, over the course of a few days, your plugged duct does not resolve, call your doctor. This can turn into mastitis, which is an infection of the breast. If you are worried in general, call your doctor.

Mastitis

The culprit of my own mastitis was a plugged duct that I did not realize I had. When you become a mother of twins, it's hard to find time for yourself or your health. You may have symptoms, but you have to take care of so many other people and things like housework that you don't notice your own discomfort. In my case, yes, I knew that I had a lump on my breast, so I tried to rub it out in the shower. No big deal. After a few days, however, the lump was still there and became red and hot to the touch. In fact, I had been feeling crappy overall.

I had felt tired (more than usual), and I felt like a bus hit me. I thought I might have had a fever, so I took the time to take my temperature. (It was nice to take a temperature that didn't have to be done rectally!) And sure enough, I had a fever. I then became engorged on the left side and entire bottom portion of my breast where the lump had been, so I called my OB-GYN's office. They had me come right in.

I officially had mastitis, and I was told to go home and let my babies nurse! I was also told to get my breast into a hot shower, allowing the hot water to hit my breast while I massaged out the pain. Warm washcloth compresses also helped. And in a few days, I was better. I had a prescription for an antibiotic if my fever didn't break within 24 hours, but my fever subsided with acetaminophen so I never needed the antibiotic. It was my doctor's philosophy that you should only take the antibiotic as a last resort (if symptoms didn't ease up in two days and fever didn't normalize in one day) since it would definitely pass into breastmilk.

If you feel engorged or lumpy along with flu-like symptoms (muscle aches, fever, a rapid pulse, and fatigue) and have a warm, red breast, you may have mastitis, which is an infection of the breast that can worsen. If you think you have mastitis, get to your doctor's office and keep breastfeeding frequently. Ask your physician if you need an antibiotic or if you should try other remedies since antibiotics pass into breastmilk. And to help ease your mind about mastitis, it is not nearly as painful as thrush. If you've had thrush, mastitis will be much less painful to get through!

Problems with Nipple Shape

If you believe you have inverted, flat, or very large nipples, ask your OB-GYN for a true diagnosis and recommendations while still pregnant. Also seek the help of a great lactation consultant before the babies arrive for best success with breastfeeding. Avoid nipple stimulation, however, before the babies are born since nipple stimulation can lead to uterine contractions and pre-term labor.

Biting

My number one fear during pregnancy and my early lactating days was biting by new, little, sharp teeth! Since I have such sensitive nipples, I just assumed that I would need to stop nursing when my babies got teeth. Other breastfeeding moms told me about biting, and I decided that I would not tolerate biting!

And then I became a seasoned, experienced, breastfeeding mom. I loved breastfeeding so much that nothing would stop me. Nothing. I decided pretty early on that I would breastfeed until my babies hit the one-year mark for sure, and I would continue beyond one year as long as my babies wanted. If my babies wanted to self-wean before their first birthday, then I would pump milk. I decided that I would do anything and everything to give my babies breastmilk.

I got past my fear of biting. It was pretty easy, actually, because my babies didn't have teeth. Even when they were teething, nothing seemed to be happening. I lived in denial that my babies would someday get teeth and perhaps try to bite.

And then Julia's first tooth popped through. Have I mentioned yet that Julia is my sassier child? If someone were going to bite, I would think Julia would be the offender. And she was! Who knew such a short tooth could hurt so much! It didn't hurt like engorgement or thrush or even childbirth, but it was unpleasant. I also thought that the bite would last a moment; however, when babies bite, they hang on. The bite lasts a minute until you yelp and let them know that it is not okay to bite.

My baby girl got the first tooth and made the first (and second) bite mark on Mommy's nipple. And yes, I did bleed from the center of my nipple (which is rare when compared to other mom friends' biting stories). As I mentioned, I yelped and said "No, No bite!" which Julia understood very well. A few minutes later, my apprehensive nipple went back into her mouth, and she thought she'd try another bite. I gave a firm, louder "NO" once again, and she literally jumped off my nursing pillow. She never tried it again!

David, on the other hand, never even thought of biting me. I think he liked eating too much to stop and bite. This brings me to a very important point. Your babies cannot bite and eat at the same time since their tongues cover their teeth while they are actively breastfeeding. If baby bites, he is playing, not eating. You should remove him from the breast promptly, tell him "NO," and give him a break. If after the break your baby still "plays" with your nipple or bites, give him another break or stop nursing him, as he may be bored or full. He will get the point quickly! Either eat or get off the breast! And then your babies will know that when they are at your breasts, you mean business!

When Your Babies are Sick

Here is a helpful tip from my great lactation consultant, Shellie: When your babies are sick with a cold or another illness, be sure to gently clean your nipples after breastfeeding to prevent spreading illness to both babies. The procedure:

1. Pat your nipples with a wet washcloth after every feeding.
2. Then squirt some breastmilk onto each nipple.
3. Let your nipples air dry.

Finally, please do not fear breastfeeding because of what could possibly happen. Many women breastfeed for more than a year and experience none of these aforementioned "pains." If you do experience any of these, I hope my descriptions, tips, and encouragement help you through the painful times. Remember, the pain is temporary. Your babies need your breastmilk, so do everything you can to get better. Get through each day, knowing that this too shall pass.

Chapter 10:
Feeling Rejected?
Nipple Confusion & Nursing Strikes

Nipple Confusion

Despite what some medical practitioners believe, I can attest that nipple confusion is real! It's so funny...I was a breastfeeding novice in the NICU, trying to get two tiny babies to my two breasts. Julia was crying at the sight of my breast, and all she wanted was that bottle that released the milk so quickly for her. I said to the nurse, "Any tips for nipple confusion?" She sharply responded, "There's no such thing as nipple confusion!" Guess what, mean nurse: **Nipple confusion is real!**

It all started when my babies were born. They were six weeks early and whisked off to the nursery for a myriad of tests after I delivered them vaginally. They also needed some time in the isolette, or warmer, to achieve an appropriate temperature since babies at low birth weights don't have enough brown fat (the fat that helps them regulate their body temperatures). While in the warmer, a nurse came into my room and told me that my babies needed nutrition to grow and get better temperature control. She told me that she needed to give them formula, so I, the dietitian that I am, freaked out. I accepted this fact, but I also demanded a pump.

Well, the nurse showed up with a single pump, perhaps thinking I wasn't serious. I called for my great lactation consultant and she got me the attachments to double pump my breasts. It was my goal to get my milk to come in, so I pumped every three hours around the clock.

My babies did try one feeding individually, and both latched well. I nursed both babies individually, and then I pumped. And I pumped in between feedings. I was GOING to do this! I don't truly remember exactly when my milk came in; however, I do remember that by the second day, I was taking teaspoonfuls of colostrum back to the nursery to be given to my babies. I kept nursing as often as possible, and my babies were getting 15-30 cc bottles of formula or formula mixed with colostrum/breastmilk. When my milk fully came in, I filled that fridge in the nursery with my wonderful breastmilk.

At that point, my babies no longer needed formula at all. Instead, they got 15-30 cc of breastmilk fortified with human milk fortifier (for extra nutrition, vitamins, and minerals) after each feeding. And by the second day, my babies' body temperatures had regulated, so they were now able to room in with my husband and me.

Everything was going well. My babies were taking the breast and latching well, but Julia started showing a preference for the bottle since it spilled breastmilk into her mouth more quickly than breastfeeding. She didn't like waiting for my let down, and she would begin to cry terribly. She began to hate my breast. And after a week, my babies were discharged from the hospital. I didn't know what to do as my daughter's disgust for my breast continued to worsen. She just loved those bottles. This was nipple confusion!

I went to a breastfeeding clinic, talked to my great lactation consultant, and cried a few times. None of these attempts at figuring out how to stop the nipple confusion worked; so I got creative. My pediatrician told me that we needed the supplemental bottles of fortified breastmilk until the babies hit six pounds. Having a Master's Degree in Counseling and a pretty good understanding of behavior change, I decided to "make" Julia like my breast with gentle trickery. I did this by giving the 30 cc supplemental bottle (only 1 ounce) of fortified breastmilk *first*, and then I would breastfeed as "dessert." The pediatrician said that I wouldn't need to give more than 30 cc of supplemental breastmilk; but as Julia's needs grew, my breastmilk supply would grow and thus be *more satisfying* than the bottle.

I gave the bottle, and my somewhat satisfied baby happily tried the breast for "dessert" since she was no longer ravenous. And sure enough, eventually that 30 cc bottle seemed like a much smaller quantity when compared to what my breasts were providing! By the six-pound mark, Julia didn't even miss losing that supplemental bottle and became a professional breastfeeder!

The moral of this story is that nipple confusion is real and is sometimes not preventable (if your babies need supplemental fortified bottles of breastmilk). What I would suggest:

✓ Make sure supplements are given with an orthodontic nipple. (Lactation consultants may want to show you how to use other ways of feeding supplemental milk like using a small syringe; however, this can be very tedious! You have TWO babies to feed! Consider this: orthodontic nipple bottles are okay to use.)

✓ Sometimes it helps to have someone else give the supplement so that baby associates you as the "breastfeeding mom" and not as the "bottle feeder."

✓ Don't give pacifiers until the babies are six to eight weeks old or when breastfeeding is well established (e.g., latching well, growing, etc.).

✓ Get support and suggestions from your pediatrician, lactation consultant, a breastfeeding clinic, or the La Leche League.

✓ Be creative...you know your babies best and may know of a trick that may get your nipple-confused baby beyond this!

✓ Don't lose faith in the process. You are much more appealing than a rubber nipple on a bottle. Keep at it to give your baby the chance to come around.

Nursing Strikes

Nursing strikes are nothing short of frustrating and annoying. In fact, nursing strikes were one of the few things that made me consider quitting breastfeeding. These are strong words coming from me, the "Type A," breastfeeding crusader that I am! But nursing strikes can bring you down! Here's what nursing strikes look like:

✓ Your babies refuse the breast.

✓ Your babies try to roll around or get away from you while you are trying to nurse.

✓ Your babies "raspberry" your nipple, blow on it, or spit milk on it.

✓ Your babies play with each other instead of nursing, pull each other's hair, poke each other's eyes, etc.

I also have a few hypotheses as to why babies "strike:"

✓ You may have waited too long to feed them.

✓ Their environment has too many distractions including people walking into the room, people talking to you, or excessive noise.

✓ You may be in unfamiliar surroundings.

✓ You may be in the presence of family your babies love, or there may be toys on the floor that your babies want to see.

✓ Your babies are overly tired and off their routine.

✓ You're on the phone.

✓ You're wearing a new perfume, deodorant, or lotion.

✓ Your babies may be teething or getting sick.

✓ Your babies may have hurt feelings or may have had a bad experience at the breast (Rosenthal & Arsenault, 2001).

✓ The babies are becoming independent and would rather be trying out a new skill.

✓ The babies simply may not be hungry since you may have added or increased their solids.

✓ You may also need to nurse less often as you add more solids and as they get older. Ask your pediatrician how many feedings they should be taking per day for their age.

Therefore, to keep nursing strikes to a minimum:

1. Nurse the babies promptly when they show signs of hunger or when they are sleepy.

2. Try to keep babies on a sleep and solids routine as best as possible so as not to disturb their body clocks, which are affected by mealtimes and sleeping times.

3. Keep your surroundings free from too much distraction while nursing.

4. Don't talk to others or talk on the phone while nursing. This is your babies' special time with you.

5. If you keep a radio or TV on while nursing, keep the volume low.

6. If you are away from home, go and nurse alone in a quiet place away from all the action. When out at a mall or shopping center, you can easily nurse in your car. (See Chapter 13 on Breastfeeding Outside Your Home.)

7. Respectfully ask that others leave the three of you alone to breastfeed.

8. Ask your spouse not to barge in while you are nursing.

9. Keep in mind that babies' nursing needs change as they get older and eat increased quantities of solid foods. Ask your pediatrician for recommendations.

10. Comfort babies with hurt feelings by showing them plenty of love and attention.

11. Don't try new deodorant, lotion, or perfume scents. You babies like your natural smell best.

12. Keep this in mind: Your babies may just be teething or wanting to do something else. If so, attempt to put them to the breast about three times before stopping nursing. To keep your milk supply adequate, you can pump at these times when your babies have not nursed well. And you will find that your babies will come to the next feeding with huge hunger and a wide-open mouth!

Chapter 11:
Pumping Through Each Stage

When to Pump at Each Stage

Talk to your lactation consultant or pediatrician about when and how often you should pump if you need to give supplemental fortified breastmilk to your babies. Otherwise, in the beginning, pump after all feedings for 15 minutes to build up your milk supply in both your breasts and to get a good supply in your freezer, especially if you plan on returning to work and will need milk for bottles. In addition, pump for 15 minutes when you need to be away from your babies, as if it were an actual feeding.

Some Facts about Pumping:
✓ One breast will generally appear to make more milk when pumping. This is normal!

✓ Let down while pumping causes a big spray followed by lots of dripping. You may need to fill up your containers, empty them into storage containers, and then continue pumping since you have so much milk!

✓ Pumping can be boring. Instead of staring at a clock, read a book, watch TV (I watched "Jeopardy®" while pumping), or listen to relaxing music.

✓ You can sleep lightly or rest your eyes while pumping, but you need to be upright and need to keep holding your containers. Don't spill your milk! (And don't cry over spilled milk! It's bound to happen at least once!)

Over time, you may notice that you are pumping less breastmilk. This occurs when your babies become more efficient and drink most of your milk. At this point, discuss with your pediatrician or lactation consultant how often you should pump. The milk I was getting from pumping significantly decreased when my babies were six weeks old. As per the advice of our pediatrician, I then pumped after every other feeding, which allowed me to rest more. Then, by eight weeks old, my pediatrician told me to wean off pumping since I had become a " normal breastfeeding mom." She told me that I could pump when I wanted (which works better in the morning when your milk supply is at its best) to gain extra milk for my freezer supply.

I also bought a deep freezer for storing breastmilk, which can extend shelf life to five to six months! And if I no longer felt like pumping, I didn't have to! All I needed to do was let my babies suckle and take my milk, and this alone kept my milk supply where it needed to be!

If you are returning to work, discuss when to pump with a lactation consultant or your babies' pediatrician to keep up a good milk supply. Know that the more you empty your breasts, the more milk you will make. Pumping will need to become an essential part of your workday!

Sometimes while pumping, I felt like I was "running out of milk" or not having a let down, but my babies continued to grow appropriately and had appropriate amounts of wet and dirty diapers. They were getting enough from my breasts! They just became very efficient (more so than the pump!). Although my breasts felt soft, my babies were suckling as much as they needed, thus telling my body how much breastmilk to make.

I did discover, however, that I had more milk in the morning (since my babies seemed to choke on my let-down), after sleeping through the night. When my babies were about seven months old, I tried pumping at night after their bedtime in an effort to replenish the supply of milk in my freezer. However, I couldn't get much milk...I realized I was tired, and my breasts had worked hard all day long. Instead, I discovered that pumping after the first morning feed around the same time each day, a good one and a half or two hours before their next feeding, worked best in getting baggies of milk back into my freezer.

Some Additional Tips:

✓ Get a hospital grade or an electric double pump...you need breastmilk for two people and need the best and most efficient products! (I started with a rented pump and then used an electric double pump.)

✓ Since you will be pumping A LOT in those beginning days, set up a pumping station in your home in a quiet place with a TV, radio, or something else to entertain you. (I still think of pumping every time I see "Jeopardy®.")

✓ Have pitchers of water at your pumping station and be sure to drink well during and after pumping.

✓ Have tissues at your pumping station to wipe up excess milk on your breasts. Let your nipples air dry. If experiencing any soreness, express some breastmilk as medicine and rub it onto your nipples. Also apply Lansinoh® regularly.

✓ Use a double pump, and pump for 15 minutes. Your milk will drip at first, and then spray after letdown (Rosenthal & Arsenault, 2001).

✓ Moisten your breasts before pumping to improve suction, and select a nipple adaptor if needed (Rosenthal & Arsenault, 2001).

✓ Learn to sleep (sitting up!) or rest while you pump.

✓ Relax!!!!

✓ Remember, the babies' suckling is ALWAYS more efficient that the pump – Don't get scared when the number of ounces on the container doesn't seem like much (Rosenthal & Arsenault, 2001).

✓ Pumping should NOT be painful!

✓ Clean your pump and attachments regularly according to the instructions.

✓ For breastmilk storage safety, remember the rule of "fives:"

Breastmilk is Safe for:
− **5 hours at room temperature**   − **5 days in the fridge**   − **5 months in the deep freezer**   **(as far away from the door as possible)**

✓ You can easily store breastmilk in ice cube trays (that have been run through the dishwasher [on the top rack] before the first use to sterilize them). Each cube is close to one ounce. Then put the cubes into a breastmilk bag, a vacuum-sealed bag, or a high quality, double bagged, zip-lock bag. *Be sure to date your bags!*

✓ Don't freeze breastmilk right after pumping – Put it in the fridge first to cool it down, and then freeze it (Rosenthal & Arsenault, 2001). It is safe to pour cooled milk onto previously frozen milk (Rosenthal & Arsenault, 2001).

✓ If you will need the milk for supplements, pour it immediately into your bottles and date them with a sharpie marker, which can be removed with rubbing alcohol or even dish soap.

✓ Thaw breastmilk under warm water or in a dish of warm water, **NEVER** in the microwave, as this will destroy many of the good properties of breastmilk and can burn the babies.

✓ Don't refreeze thawed milk, and use it within 24 hours (AAP, 2004).

✓ Thawed breastmilk may be different colors based on your varied diet and separates into milk and cream, so just shake it up well before serving (Rosenthal & Arsenault, 2001).

Pumping Hygiene

In the hospital, the nurses told me to "just rinse out the containers and pump parts with hot water." To me, this sounded unsanitary, and it *was!* AAP (2004) recommends the following for good hygiene:

✓ Bicycle-horn type pumps should not be used since these can become very contaminated.

✓ Clean collection containers and pump parts in hot soapy water, and let them air-dry.

✓ If dishwasher safe, you may use the dishwasher also.

✓ Follow the storage breastmilk tips as mentioned ("the rule of fives").

Going Back to Work

Although I did not return to work for quite some time, I would still like to provide tips from successful breastfeeding working mothers and professionals so you can continue to give your twins the best source of nutrition. Breastfeeding twins is challenging to begin with; returning to work and continuing to give your twins breastmilk can be even harder. Many women, however, are very successful in providing breastmilk for their twin babies despite returning to work. All it takes is support and planning:

✓ Take as much time off as you can or take a Family Medical Leave of Absence so that you can get breastfeeding well established (for at least the first six to eight weeks).

✓ Wait until your babies are four to six weeks old to introduce a bottle to avoid nipple confusion, and have your spouse or another family member introduce bottles of breastmilk to enhance their acceptance of the bottle when you return to work.

✓ Talk to your boss, co-workers, and human resources department about your decision to breastfeed your twins.

✓ Explain to your workplace that breastfeeding your twins will make you a better employee in that you will need less time off when your babies get sick since they will be receiving the immune-enhancing properties of breastmilk.

✓ Be sure to use a good, double pump to cut down on the time it takes to pump.

✓ Bring pieces of the babies' clothing, relaxing music, and/or the babies' photos so that you can let down and get a good quantity of milk.

✓ Tell your bosses that you need one to two 15-minute breaks per eight hours to pump, and request a clean, quiet, comfortable, and private location for pumping. This can include an executive's office, for example, during their lunch break.

✓ Date your milk, place it in a zip lock bag, and keep it in a refrigerator or in a cooler with an ice pack.

✓ Invest in blouses or shirts that can easily be maneuvered for pumping at work.

✓ If you live close to work or if the daycare is close to your workplace, go to your babies for a breastfeeding session.

✓ Have your babies meet their caretaker or day care staff ahead of time to enhance their acceptance of this new setting.

Chapter 12:
Yours, His, or Theirs?

Sexual Objects AND Feeding Devices?

For those women who do not yet have children, their breasts are their own and are sometimes shared with a spouse or partner for sexual purposes. Many men in committed relationships then view their partner's breasts as objects for *their own* sexual pleasure. But, after birthing not one, but two (or more) babies... your two milky breasts seem to belong solely to those two hungry babies!

Well, this leaves little or no time for your spouse. He may feel left out or even rejected since he is no longer getting "breast time" whenever he wants. The novelty of having them at his disposal is now gone.

Then, you may even start to feel like the babies are at your breasts so much, suckling and tugging away, that they are no longer even YOURS! This sounds weird, mainly because it's truly YOUR body. But you lose control over your breasts. Their main function becomes feeding your babies, and you may feel as though you have lost this part of your body for the time being.

For me, I felt like my breasts were my bottles, my feeding devices, and my source of nourishment for the babies (their ONLY source of nourishment). My breasts were no longer mine, and they were definitely no longer my husband's. They were NOT sexual; in fact, I had to finally work up the nerve to tell my husband to stay away. I felt like he was desecrating my feeding devices. He was making my pure nutrition impure by going anywhere near my breasts, which now were dedicated to my children only.

I felt guilty about feeling this way, but then I learned that many other breastfeeding mothers also feel as though their breasts are for their babies only. If you are having these same feelings, you are COMPLETELY normal. Once you stop breastfeeding, your breasts can return to their previous roles/functions. If, on the other hand, you are feeling resentful about all this, remember that breastfeeding is the best thing you can do for your babies and that it is only a temporary experience.

Keep Connected With Your Spouse

There are many ways you can creatively keep connected with your spouse. Use the following tips to re-connect!

For Example:

✓   Tell your spouse you love him daily.

✓   Don't forget to snuggle, cuddle, hold hands, and hug and kiss. Sometimes these can be great replacements instead of that "tired lovemaking."

✓   Have "date night" after the babies go to bed. Enjoy a meal and watch a movie together at home after bedtime.

✓   Do kind things for your spouse like making his lunch or making his favorite dinner on occasion.

✓   When your spouse does nice things for you or offers additional help beyond his norm, be sure to thank him.

✓   Make love during naptimes.

Things You Can't Control About Your Breasts

Leaking!
I wish someone had told me about leaking. In the beginning, when your milk finally comes in after two days or so, your breasts leak A LOT! A friend of mine never wore a bra and just leaked all over her t-shirts; however, I couldn't stand feeling wet. To make leaking more manageable, use breast pads regularly.

    I found it better to use the disposable breast pads for outings, and you can then easily bring plenty of extras in your diaper bag to toss in the trash when you've finished using them. At home, I used overnight breast pads (better absorption) faithfully. I didn't typically use these in public unless I had run out of disposables because I found that two blatant circles showed right through my shirt, screaming BREAST PADS UNDER HERE!

    It's also a good idea to use Lansinoh® or another lanolin cream from the start to prevent having sore or cracked nipples (which can make or break your breastfeeding experience). But an important thing I learned about lanolin is that it stains terribly and doesn't come out, even with stain removers! Definitely use disposable breast pads when using lanolin creams to protect your bra and clothing!

    Then one day, you just stop needing lanolin cream. And then a few months later, you just stop leaking. I don't remember exactly when I stopped leaking because I kept wearing breast pads for fear of leaking through my tops.

But somewhere around the three-month mark, I remember I stopped using breast pads since I had not leaked in quite a while. It was a liberating time, and it made getting the babies to my breasts a quicker task. It also felt good to finally be nice and dry...no stickiness and no itchiness!

I thought I was finally in the clear with leaking, and then the babies started sleeping through the night at five months old. Granted, it was wonderful to be able to sleep through the night, but it caused all kinds of problems for my breasts (See Chapter 19). Sleeping through the night also caused my breasts to start leaking again! Who knew!

It made sense...the time between feedings was longer since the babies were sleeping through the night. The longer the span, the more time milk has to fill up in your breasts. This leads to engorgement, which then leads to leaking. For about one month after the babies started sleeping through the night, I leaked like crazy at night! My breast pads were swollen with milk! Sometimes I even contemplated wringing them out and saving the milk (just kidding, don't do this!). Finally, around seven months, my overnight leakage became scant or sometimes even nonexistent. But I had to mention this phenomenon...No one else remembers to tell you what sleeping through the night (such a wonderful event) does to your breasts!

The Trick to Stop Leaking on the Spot

As I've mentioned earlier, remember your teenage days when you would go to a pool or to the beach? Remember when the cold wind would come by just after you got out of the water? And remember how your nipples got erect and showed through your swimsuit, which was very embarrassing? What did you do? You more than likely put your forearms up against your nipples gently to warm yourself and make your nipples return to their normal appearance. This same technique, **whereby you take your forearms and gently hold them against your nipples**, also stops leaking on the spot. Just make sure you always have breast pads on or in your bag. If you forget them, use some tissue or toilet paper!

Sagging Breasts!

In addition, my lactation consultant told me that if I didn't wear a bra ALL THE TIME (even while sleeping) that my breasts would become a saggy mess. I immediately put on a soft, non-underwire nursing bra or sports bra that buttoned down the front, and I've never removed a bra since (besides for showers!). All in all, I found that wearing a bra all the time was truly more comfortable and that using breast pads was a must!

Regarding breast changes, breast size, or sagging, there is no solid research on what is normal. After nursing, some women sag, while others stay perky. Always wear a bra to better your chances of perkiness. In addition, some women keep their large, milky looking breasts, and other women's breasts seem to disappear. Anything goes in regard to post-lactation breast changes! There is no norm! However, if you notice anything strange to include lumps or other breast changes, immediately consult your OB-GYN.

Chapter 13:
When Others May See Your Boobs:
Successfully Breastfeeding Twins Outside Your Home

The thought of breastfeeding two babies outside your home and without your loveseat can be daunting. But I promise you: This can be done modestly and successfully. One thing you need to know upfront, however, is that you will always need a nursing pillow to nurse outside the home successfully. And luckily, one will definitely fit in the base of a double stroller! It is also extremely helpful to have a helper!

Going out for a Short Time

If you want to run to one store or go out for a quick meal, plan your trip according to your babies and when they usually nurse. Then, you can nurse them immediately before you leave. Also, have the babies totally dressed and ready prior to nursing so that you have enough time to run your errand or do your shopping prior to the next feeding. Once they stop suckling from one feeding, the clock starts ticking until the time when they will become hungry again. So nurse and go! I remember planning all of my grocery trips this way, and I even went to a church service around the time my babies nursed.

It is okay to breastfeed in public! (For breastfeeding "in public" support, see: www.nurseherenow.com.) However, breastfeeding before leaving the house is comfortable since you have your loveseat or large chair, and it is more practical when you will not be bringing a helper along.

When breastfeeding twins in public, three main issues can potentially arise: the babies can become distracted and not feed well (also known as a nursing strike), the Mommy may feel awkward or stressed (which makes it difficult to let down), and there may be a lack of comfort in locations other than the home. If you can help it, do your best to pre-plan and pre-event breastfeed for ultimate comfort and a good quality feeding. However...

If you have no control over the timing of an event like an appointment or a party, then you can do your best to nurse before you leave the house. If you cannot nurse prior to leaving your home, then make sure you bring a helper along. Read on for more tips on nursing twins in places other than your home.

Going out for Extended Periods of Time

If you don't have control over the time of an event and your babies cannot nurse before you leave the house or if your are going out for an extended period of time, you can do the following:

✓ Absolutely bring your nursing pillow.

✓ Absolutely bring a partner to help you. If you are going to a place alone, be sure there will be someone there to help you. The helper can assist with modesty by standing in front of your breasts while getting both babies latched (the timeframe where both breasts can potentially be exposed), by handing you each baby, and by providing support and the "eye" for people who might be overtly glaring at you!

✓ If you are going to a party or someone's home, find a quiet place to nurse that is away from the action so that the babies can focus. Use a loveseat or the side of a bed. If you use the side of a bed, it helps to prop your feet onto something.

✓ If you will be out shopping for the day or going out of town, you can nurse in the backseat of a car comfortably since there is extra space.

- Nursing while in *your* car is okay! Ignore people's glares or stares!

- Still self-conscious that you might bare both breasts in public? Remember all those receiving blankets you got at your shower? Sit in the passenger seat and roll down the window slightly so that you can put one over the window for modesty. Roll the window back up and you will have a nice shade. You can hang another receiving blanket or two from the visors, and you'll have a good amount of quick privacy.

- If you have a vehicle with a third row seat, you can easily nurse in the third row without anyone even knowing what you are doing back there.

✓ If you don't want to nurse in a car, you can easily find a bench or other chair. Benches are more comfortable if they have "backs."

✓ Once seated comfortably, have your partner hand you both babies. Then, you can have your partner hold up a receiving blanket while you unleash both breasts for both babies (In many states, you are breaking NO laws by breastfeeding in public so your babies can eat—see more below*).

✓ If you are shopping and there is a dressing room or comfortable sitting area or lounge with couches, this works very well!

✓ Breastfeeding in public is now legal in many states. (*You can check the La Leche League website or your state's website for more information on the legal status of breastfeeding in public in your state.) I've nursed in public many times at birthday parties, family gatherings, parks, outings, Disney World, malls, etc., and the most people see is two small bobbing heads!

✓ If you do desire privacy when breastfeeding in public, you can take your chair to the corner of the room and face the wall. This also helps the babies to keep focused and not get as distracted.

✓ Finally, remember this: When breastfeeding in public, someone is likely to say the following: *"Why don't you go to a bathroom to do that?"* A possible response: *"Would you eat your dinner in a public restroom?"*

Going to Disney World (or Similar Places) for the Day

If you will be out for the entire day, you can use many of the tips I've mentioned. I found that parks or similar places do have private areas or even first aid stations that will accommodate breastfeeding mothers. You can ask to use a rest area or lounge, or you can ask to borrow an office. Be creative to achieve the most relaxing and comfortable breastfeeding experience while out for the whole day. And if you need to use that park bench, it can be done! Trust me!

Traveling

Traveling can also pose some breastfeeding difficulty when you have to nurse two babies. As I've already recommended, definitely nurse your babies before you leave the house. If you are getting on a plane, train, or bus, consider nursing them again in the parking lot or in a quiet seating area before you leave since the seating tends to be tight on these modes of transportation.

You can plan your seating ahead of time too. For example, it may be wise to sit in the last row with your spouse across from you for extra space if you need to nurse while en route. As a special note, airlines prohibit two lap babies in the same section since there are only four oxygen masks per three-seat section (only one extra mask pops out overhead for each section). Therefore, only one lap baby is allowed per seating section. When making travel arrangements, choose a seat across from your spouse in the same row instead.

Also, remember that the changes in air pressure may affect your babies by causing them ear discomfort. It helps to let them suck while ascending and descending, so make sure they are awake and provide them with something for sucking (your breasts, a bottle of breastmilk, a pacifier, or a sippy cup of water).

I discovered a few more breastfeeding traveling tips when my husband and I flew to Florida when my babies were three months old:

✓ I brought a small cooler of iced-down, pumped milk for the plane, just in case I needed an unlimited quantity of breastmilk and didn't have the space to nurse.

✓ I brought a battery-operated breast pump in the diaper bag in case of needing milk at an awkward time. I figured I could pump in a bathroom if need be.

✓ A nursing pillow fit in my husband's backpack – great for "layover nursing."

✓ In the airport, I found a secluded spot in the waiting areas for breastfeeding. My husband and sister held blankets for privacy while I latched the babies.

✓ If people got too close or began to stare, my husband gave them the "eye."

Other Twin Travel Tips:

✓ A play yard fits into a large duffle bag and can be checked as a carry-on item when flying. (Or it can be checked in its original case.)

✓ Double strollers that hold your infant car seats can typically be checked at the gate for free. Your car seats can then be checked along with the stroller for free!

✓ Limit the number of hotel or location transfers…each change requires your babies to adjust to their new environment, and they may become frustrated.

✓ Bring dusk-to-dawn nightlights to make your babies feel safe and secure in their sleeping areas.

✓ Continue your routine as closely as possible, but also be flexible. Your babies may need to nap in your arms if you are out, or you may need to skip a nap. Just return to your routine the next day.

✓ Bring a Boppy® cover so that your nursing pillow is protected.

✓ Expect some nursing strikes since your babies will be in different surroundings and around different people.

✓ If your babies will not nurse for a particular feeding, be sure to pump your breasts or manually express as much milk as possible to keep your milk supply at its best.

✓ Put a "do not disturb" sign on your hotel room during naptime! You wouldn't believe how hard it is to get a housekeeper out of the room even once she realizes you have twin babies who are trying to sleep!

✓ Use disinfecting wipes to spruce up the hotel room. If your babies are crawling, consider asking the lobby staff for a vacuum to spruce up the floors.

✓ Bring your own tub mat to prevent slipping during bath time.

✓ If traveling by car, find a large parking lot and use my aforementioned car breastfeeding method if you want modesty.

✓ Please note that car trips will take much, much longer than usual when adding in breastfeeding time. My seven-hour drive from Virginia to Pennsylvania ended up taking 10 hours! Plan ahead by leaving earlier or by breaking the trip up with a hotel stay.

✓ Travel is more difficult with children, as you need to pre-plan, pack everything under the sun, and think ahead about everything; however, vacations with children are filled with so much laughter and joy! It's worth every bit of planning!

Read on for a great travel checklist!

HERE IS A TRAVELING CHECKLIST TO USE BEFORE EACH TRIP:

For the plane:	*For the hotel / vacation:*
✓ Large backpack that will fit your nursing pillow ✓ Nursing pillow ✓ Pacifiers (after eight weeks, if you use them, since sucking can reduce pressure in their ears while flying – Breastfeeding can do the same thing!) ✓ Toys, book, musical toys ✓ Battery operated/plug-in type pump ✓ Bottles of thawed breastmilk in a cooler with an icepack ✓ Sippy cups, food, snacks, etc. for older babies ✓ Big bottle of water and snacks for you ✓ Diaper bag with extra diapers, wipes, clothes/pajamas, onesies, socks, bibs ✓ Oversized changing pad ✓ Disposable bibs ✓ Medicines, acetaminophen, ibuprofen, baby vitamins ✓ Double stroller with infant seats (if still in these) ✓ Blankets ✓ Watch, cell phone, charger for cell phone ✓ Tissues, hand sanitizer, extra disinfecting wipes ✓ Small disposal baggies for diapers, dirty bibs or feeding supplies, trash, or dirty clothing ✓ Feeding logs so you remember who goes where, who pooped last, and when the last feeding was	✓ Battery operated/plug-in type pump ✓ 1-2 play yards (depending on ages, sizes, and sleep habits of babies) ✓ Folding dining chairs ✓ Plates, bowls, utensils, cups, bibs, disposable bibs ✓ Food, diapers and wipes (Can also be purchased at end location if in the U.S.) ✓ Medicines, acetaminophen, ibuprofen, baby vitamins ✓ Baby monitors ✓ Small radio to make it "day" during naps (if no alarm clock in room) ✓ Nightlights ✓ Thermometer, nail clippers, bulb syringes ✓ Other regularly used toiletries, lotions, creams ✓ Sunscreen, hats, sunglasses, swimwear, swim diapers ✓ Bath supplies to include non-skid bath mat, body wash, towels, wash cloths, lotions, bath toys ✓ Coats, hats, sweaters/sweatshirts ✓ Onesies, socks, clothes plus extras, pajamas plus extras, shoes ✓ Breast pads and plenty of nursing bras ✓ Camera/video camera, charging equipment ✓ Journal

Chapter 14:
Fashion Tips for Moms of Twins
...Keeping "Boobs" in Mind!

Although I'm no fashion diva, I did like to keep up-to-date with fashion despite being a breastfeeding mother of twins. I just found those breastfeeding clothes nauseating, and they really don't work for twins since you need both breasts exposed. I'll share with you what I learned about fashion and nursing twins:

✓ Immediately after the twins were born, people told me to "just wear my maternity clothes." YUCK! I didn't want to wear these! I searched my closet for larger clothing, and I hit some yard sales for cheap, stylish, in-between clothing! (You can also go to stores like Wal-Mart® or Target® and hit the sales racks for transition clothes!)

✓ As for tops, breastfeeding-type clothing and button down blouses do not work. You need both breasts exposed!

✓ Believe it or not, tighter tops work great because you can pull them up above your breasts and they stay up. This prevents clothing from interfering with nursing and keeps part of you covered.

✓ Considering buying those new breastfeeding tops with a built in bra top and two holes underneath? These tops are not so great if you're nursing two babies. You essentially end up showing everyone your breasts through the two peek holes since you need to expose both breasts to feed both babies.

✓ Sports bras that button up the front, on the other hand, are awesome! All you have to do is lift these up above your breasts to nurse! Also, they work great for nighttime support. (I am actually wearing this type of bra in the photos in Chapter 3.)

✓ NEVER use nursing bras with underwires!

✓ Dresses do not work unless they have stretchy straps or no straps. And if you have no straps or stretchy straps, you have to take your top down, which is a lot more risqué than pulling your top up. (And more risqué since your babies can easily disrobe you!)

✓ Silky pajama bottoms cannot support a nursing pillow...your babies will slide right off. Stick to cotton pajamas!

✓ As for jewelry, I found that it either interfered with nursing since it was distracting or it ended up being pulled (which hurts)...although some moms swear by using a beaded necklace for "bored" seven-month old breastfeeders to keep them occupied!

✓ About hair: I actually grew mine long so that I could pull it back daily. With short hair, it often needs to be styled and will still get pulled. I went with longer locks.

✓ For me, I found that very fashionable high-heeled shoes were dangerous when I was trying to manage two babies.

✓ For stay-at-home moms: Each day, be sure to shower, throw on a little makeup, and do other things to primp so you feel like a real person! In addition, put something on that isn't pajamas! Pajamas are for nighttime only (unless you are sick!). Sweatpants and t-shirts do count as outfits.

✓ Last but not least, enjoy your voluptuous self! Your breasts may never look this fantastic again! Women (like myself) who began as flat-chested, "nearly A" cups: Enjoy having bodacious and beautiful boobs! If you started out as a voluptuous woman, more power to you!

✓ Regardless of how you started or where you are now, celebrate yourself and celebrate motherhood by adorning and praising your beautiful and strong "mommy" body!

Part III:

What I Did and What I Learned

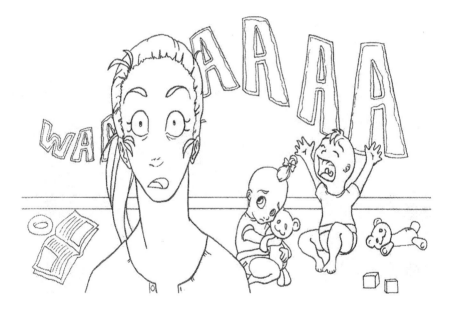

Chapter 15:
My Twin Labor Experience

During my uneventful (for the most part) pregnancy, I heard so much negativity about how "hard" it is to breastfeed twins from mothers of twins, from family members, and from health professionals that I had pretty much talked myself out of breastfeeding my twins exclusively. I just thought I would have to use some formula to supplement the twins' nutrition because everyone said so. It was not until I talked to my dietitian friend, Chantaye, who had just nursed for a full year with painful rheumatoid arthritis, that I had mentally decided that I could do this. And the more people told me I couldn't nurse twins; the more I decided I **would** nurse twins solely and successfully! I had my mind set on breastfeeding no matter what! Then I went into pre-term labor at 28 weeks along.

Well, I wasn't ready for that, and I became scared about all this parenting stuff, especially the breastfeeding part. Luckily, however, I had already met a great lactation consultant prior to delivering my babies (she taught my childbirth classes), so I was ready with a great teacher and source of support even if the babies were to come this early. Fortunately, my physician was able to stop labor with terbutaline shots, and later the oral form of the drug, every four hours for five weeks. I was scared about the side effects of this drug since it's not currently approved by the Food and Drug Administration (FDA) for the purpose of stopping labor (it's an asthma drug), but it was much scarier to think about having NICU babies born weighing less than two pounds with feeding tubes and ventilators.

At 32 weeks along, however, the babies wanted to come. I went into labor (4 cm dilated and 80% effaced), and I was put on a 48-hour magnesium sulfate drip and hospital bed rest. I had a catheter placed because I was literally not allowed to leave my bed for two days, and it was just **not** fun. The magnesium sulfate caused hot flashes, blurred vision, body and muscle spasms, and numbness. While at the time this seemed like a horrific experience, it was worth it for the sake of my babies and their health.

In the meantime, I received two steroid shots (betamethasone) for the babies' lung development and about 20 internal pelvic exams to determine my effacement and dilation. I also couldn't eat or drink anything for those two days. I remember my mom kept asking the OB-GYNs at the hospital how my babies were going to grow if I wasn't eating anything! In addition, never before in my life did I just want to pee on a *toilet* (catheters are NOT fun), take a shower, eat a simple meal, and if nothing else, drink something other than ice chips!

While this may sound scary and terrible to you, I'll tell you now not to worry about any of this. While typing this section, I could barely recall this experience and had to refer to my pregnancy journal. The birth of my babies was such a miraculous and awesome experience that it literally deleted this difficult experience from my mind. What I am sharing with you is from my written "pretty" journal, rather than a memory that has stayed fresh in my mind.

After 48 hours of magnesium sulfate, I was transferred to a regular room on the maternity floor, which I named the "Hospital Inn." My great room had a big shower with a chair in it...Wish I had one of these at home for the last trimester of my twin pregnancy! Also, I had an adjustable bed, which gave me the best sleep ever! At home, I had been trying to arrange pillows so I could sleep upright and not put any additional pressure on my abdomen and surrounding muscles; however, at the hospital, I slept like a baby with the best position at all times since I could forever adjust my bed!

Then I was discharged after a four-day stay at the hospital. My labor had stopped, so I went home on strict bed rest. And within 24 hours, I went back into labor. And did I mention that I always went into labor in the middle of the night? The first time, I ran to the hospital without having showered or eaten first, and then I was not allowed to shower or eat for three days straight. This time, I ate frozen waffles with lots of syrup at 3:00 am and took a nice warm shower, not knowing what would happen this time around.

I was given more terbutaline to stop labor, and I stayed in the hospital this time for another five days. I was 5 cm dilated and 100% effaced, so the "high risk pregnancy" physicians taking care of me were sure I would labor soon. But I didn't. I was discharged again, and I saw my regular OB-GYN the day after my second hospital discharge at exactly 34 weeks along.

At 34 weeks and 2 days, I went into labor again. My OB-GYN feared that I had been effaced for so long that I might be at risk for an infection, so she admitted me to the hospital. I was also having regular contractions yet again, but my water had not broken. She broke my water and got the anesthesiologist to come in with my epidural. I didn't have a choice as to whether or not I wanted an epidural since I might need an emergency caesarian-section. If one or both twins happened to turn during labor, then the c-section would be likely. I was also taken to the Operating Room to labor just in case I needed the c-section. My epidural was great, and my labor pain was controlled well.

Throughout my pregnancy, I didn't find out the sexes of my twins, so this experience was a great surprise! Baby A was positioned vertex, which is the correct, head down position; however, Baby B was sideways or transverse. As I pushed Baby A, an operating room technician pushed on my abdomen to turn Baby B. He was successful, and my labor experience was nothing short of miraculous and amazing! It took me 45 minutes to labor Baby A, David, and then 20 minutes to labor Baby, B, Julia! I was very lucky, as many women do require c-sections to deliver their twins.

One trend I do want to mention is that OB-GYNs are now more commonly allowing women to opt for a c-section without even trying a vaginal delivery. Sometimes, they may even recommend a c-section since multiples are considered a high-risk situation. It is your decision as to whether or not you agree with this; however, do remember that a c-section is very serious surgery that comes with side effects including very sleepy and groggy babies who may not want to nurse, a very sore and tired mommy, and a wound that will take weeks to heal. **If you need a c-section for an emergency situation and the safest delivery possible, please follow your physician's advice.** However, if your labor is going well and both babies are vertex or if one can be turned like in my scenario, then you can consider trying for a vaginal birth.

Finally, I want to provide a few tips for extending your pregnancy as long as possible based on my experience and based on recommendations from the March of Dimes:

✓ Begin prenatal vitamins and abstinence from alcohol/smoking/drugs of any sort well before attempting conception.

✓ Get early and regular prenatal care.

✓ Eat well and focus on nutritious foods (See Chapter 5 for healthy eating recommendations). Also, ask your physician about the need for iron supplementation during your pregnancy. You can also ask your physician if he or she recommends a DHA supplement like Expecta® Lipil® for eye and brain development of the babies.

✓ Don't smoke or go near people who smoke.

✓ Don't drink any alcohol at all.

✓ Avoid drugs of any kind. Ask your doctor which over the counter drugs are safe during pregnancy.

✓ Take it easy at work and home, and ask your doctor about the type, amount, and safety of exercise throughout your pregnancy. Going for walks in the first trimester may be fine; but if you feel tired, limit activity. Listen to your body!

✓   In the first trimester, invest in an exercise ball instead:

-   Sit on it for 20-30 minutes nightly.

-   Practice sitting up straight (for back strength), and roll both front to back and side to side to stretch out your hips and strengthen your pelvic floor muscles.

-   You can also make it a point to do your kegal exercises while on the exercise ball (if your don't know how, ask your doctor how to do these – it's much like starting and stopping the flow of urine).

-   For those kegal exercises: Work up to 30 reps lasting one second long and 30 reps lasting 10 seconds long EVERY NIGHT so your kegals or "pushing muscles" are strong and ready to go!

-   I truly believe these exercises helped keep back pain at bay during my pregnancy and also helped me to have a vaginal delivery of my twins in less than an hour!

✓   In the last trimester, stay off your feet as much as possible. If given bed rest orders, ask what the physician means specifically. Bed rest can mean many different things to different people.

✓   If you go into preterm labor and require a hospital stay, try to stay as relaxed and calm as possible. Bring a calling card and a list of friends' phone numbers, plenty of books and magazines, photos and empty albums, a CD player and calming music, your favorite snacks, etc. so that you can remain comfortable, calm, and entertained before your twins arrive!

Chapter 16:
Time to Breastfeed Twins

The Rudat Twins Arrive!

David (Baby A) and Julia (Baby B)
arrived on June 9, 2005.
David was born at 6:01 pm, and
Julia was born at 6:21 pm.

As for their stats:
David: 4 lbs. 1 oz., 18 in. long
Julia: 4 lbs. 6 oz., 17 in. long

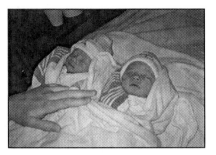

Time to Breastfeed!

I had read in many multiples books that you should get your babies to your breasts soon after they are born. This is so true! Since early breastmilk (colostrum) is so beneficial and since both mom and babies need to learn this new skill, it is imperative that you get your babies to your breasts as soon as medically possible.

Demand that your babies "room in" if medically stable so that you can breastfeed on demand when you notice hunger cues such as rooting (turning towards the breast when the cheek is touched), mouthing, increased activity or alertness, or fussiness. Crying is a late hunger signal, and having your baby near you can prevent getting to the point of hungry crying. One other tip: Make sure that you are vocal and clear about your babies breastfeeding and NOT receiving any bottles of formula (if medically stable) or pacifiers since these can lead to nipple confusion!

In reference to multiple births, I also read that you need to nurse your babies at the same time, which is true. However, when your tiny babies are just born, you and your babies need to *learn* to breastfeed, much like learning to ride a bike or drive a car; therefore, I would suggest getting the hang of nursing one baby at a time first so you know how to breastfeed in general. It is like learning any new task; it can be challenging and frustrating!

Your babies may also be different types of nursers. David immediately took the breast and latched on perfectly. He suckled strongly from the start, but he often fell asleep at the breast and needed to be awakened constantly. Julia, on the other hand, had taken a bottle in the hospital's nursery and liked how the milk in the bottle came out quickly. At that point in time, my milk had not yet come in so she became frustrated at my breast. She would cry and cry when put at my breast; she had fallen victim to nipple confusion all too soon!

In the beginning, I first had to learn how to breastfeed in general, and I had to get used to nursing two different types of nursers. By the second day, however, when I was feeling more competent. I decided to ask my great lactation consultant to show me how to tandem nurse, and from that point forward, that's how I did it. That's how I would need to do it at home, so I really wanted to get proficient at tandem nursing. And I recommend this for you also!

First, learn to nurse your very different nursers one at a time. Then, as soon as you feel comfortable with it, get them on both your breasts simultaneously or tandem with the help of another person. And you should try tandem nursing soon...don't wait too long! You will need this skill at home. Get your babies used to this type of feeding early on!

(NOTE: If there is greater than a 1 lb. difference in the size of your babies, you may need to add extra feedings for the smaller baby.)

The first few days of life with twins are a blur. You have to learn so many things about caring for two babies; and if your babies have medical issues, it can be even more complex. Since my twins were only six weeks early and I had been given two doses of steroid shots during my pre-term labor, my babies had no medical issues at birth other than immature temperature regulation. Both babies had to stay a short while in a warmer or isolette, and they needed to be double swaddled in receiving blankets for additional warmth. Because of their temperature issues and low birth weight, David and Julia required a weeklong hospital stay. And the hospital extended my stay by offering me a hospitality suite so that I could continue nursing them.

Back to the Beginning: My Babies Needed a Little Bit of Formula
For the first few hours of my babies' lives, nurses told me that they had to give formula to my babies while in the Neonatal Intensive Care Unit (NICU) to promote quick growth until my milk came in. As soon as I was rolled into a room, I requested a pump. Soon after, my great lactation consultant brought me a second set of pumping supplies so I could double pump. And I pumped and pumped and pumped with the goal of getting my milk in so my babies could get off formula. In the meantime, I delivered every drop of colostrum I collected to the nursery to be put into the bottles of formula for my babies. And when my milk came in within two days, I filled the NICU fridge with enough milk to feed all the babies there!

At that point, I told the nursing staff that I no longer wanted my babies to receive ANY formula at all. I had plenty of breastmilk in the fridge that could be fortified appropriately with human milk fortifier, which adds more nutrition to breastmilk for quicker growth. I also specifically asked the nurses to allow me to *breastfeed* my babies *first* before they provided the supplemental bottle of breastmilk. And I also specifically asked the NICU nurses NOT to use a pacifier, advice which some of them ignored. I just wanted to avoid nipple confusion as much as possible.

Learning and Troubleshooting
In those beginning days, I pretty much spent all of my time learning to breastfeed my twins. After I was asked to leave the hospitality suite of the hospital so others could use it, my babies spent an additional week at the hospital for monitoring. To ensure that my breastfeeding would continue to be successful, I went to the hospital every three hours for that week to breastfeed. I brought my sister along so she could hand me both babies, and I breastfed them as best as I could.

I also went to the hospital for nighttime feedings. I did skip one, middle-of-the-night feeding to catch up on some sleep, and the nurses gave my twins pumped milk I had provided for that particular feeding. I also made sure to ask at every shift if the babies were getting my pumped milk, and I checked the fridge myself to ensure this. It is very important to take a proactive stance with your babies' nutrition since some nurses don't care if your babies get your milk or formula.

All the while, my babies and I were constantly learning the new skill of breastfeeding. I also had to learn to troubleshoot since Julia was obviously nipple confused from the fake or artificial nipples on the supplemental bottles and from the occasional pacifiers provided by non-breastfeeding friendly nurses in the NICU. As mentioned, I'll always remember that one particular day in the NICU's breastfeeding room when a nurse informed me that there was no such thing as nipple confusion. Looking back, Julia *did* experience nipple confusion, and I cried many tears in dealing with this terrible and true phenomenon! I hope this nurse is reading, because NIPPLE CONFUSION IS REAL. It took a good two months to get over nipple confusion issues and to get Julia to accept my breast with a happy face rather than a screaming one!

Be sure to do everything possible to avoid nipple confusion like making sure your babies get only breastfeeding-friendly feeding methods if they need supplemental breastmilk (cup feeding, spoon feeding, orthodontic nipple bottles, etc.) and no pacifiers until at least six weeks old (See Chapter 18). In addition, it does help if someone other than you provides the supplemental bottle so that the babies associate you with breastfeeding and not with the bottle.

Once my babies came home from the hospital, my sister stayed with me for a whole month and handed me the babies for every feeding. I nursed on demand during the daytime, but I had to wake them every three hours overnight to get breastmilk into them to promote quick growth. After every feeding from day one, I pumped for 15 minutes to get additional milk. Also, after every feeding from day one, the babies needed a 15 to 30 cc (30 cc = one ounce) bottle (with an orthodontic nipple) of breastmilk with some human milk fortifier or premature baby formula powder added to increase the calories. If you need to do this, consult your pediatrician or dietitian for the correct mathematical formula for adding premature formula powder to breastmilk.

As mentioned, David was a better nurser, so he rejected the bottle. If I could get 15 cc of the supplemental bottle into him, it was a miracle! Julia, on the other hand, wanted the bottle and not the breast. Julia would scream at the breast, but I would make her try to nurse. I would calmly talk to her and ease her into latching on. She would suckle for a few minutes, and then she would start to scream again. When it came time for her 30 cc bottle, she would happily chug it down within five minutes! This made me cry so many times!

I was so hurt and frustrated that I called a breastfeeding help line. They said that my issue was complex and that I needed to attend a breastfeeding clinic. At the clinic, they charged me $20 and told me that I may need a supplemental nutrition system, which is a contraption that holds pumped milk in a necklace around your neck. Extending from the necklace are two tubes that attach to your nipples with tape, and this allows more milk to come out during feedings. The lactation consultant at the clinic thought this would solve the problem and sent me home with some literature and ordering information. Well, having to tape this contraption to my nipples 8 to 10 times a day and care for twins seemed like a complex, time-consuming suggestion that I was not willing to try!

I came up with my own solution...I would give Julia her 30 cc supplemental bottle *first* to get her calm, and then I would nurse her for "dessert!" Sure enough, over time, it worked! She still had her moments of breast refusal, but as my milk quantity increased and that 30 cc bottle remained the same quantity, she became more interested in my flowing, milky breast.

In addition, I always served that supplemental bottle cold or at room temperature to make the breastmilk that came from my warm breast more appealing. Over the course of two weeks or so, she was taking my breast without any hesitation. And at six weeks old, we got rid of supplemental bottles altogether since we hit the six-pound mark (which is often considered the "safe weight" by pediatricians)!

Through this experience, I discovered that the neither the breast clinic nor hotline were helpful for my issue since I needed hands-on help. (And as I mentioned earlier, not all lactation consultants are created equally.) I apprehensively pulled out my great lactation consultant's home phone number and email address. She was so thrilled to hear from me and to hear that I was still trying my hardest to breastfeed twins that she was glad to help! I would say that during the first six weeks of my twins' lives, I called and emailed her at least 10 times! And we're friends to this day! She even lent me *her* breast pump to save me money!

The moral of the story with learning to breastfeed your twins is that it may be challenging, difficult, and downright frustrating. However, use a great lactation consultant as your support person and teacher. Be creative and break rules that some pregnancy books recommend so you can get your two babies to your two breasts effectively and happily. Don't quit! It may be tough, but it's temporary. You'll get through this! Just keep trying and doing the best you can!

How Does Breastfeeding *Feel*?

I remember one thing that concerned me was the *feel* of breastfeeding. Sorry for providing too much information, but I have very sensitive nipples. Therefore, I always wondered what suckling and stretching my nipples would feel like. When I put my first baby to my breast for the first time, it simply felt like a big tug at my nipple and areola. In fact, it feels like a tug at your whole breast, but it is not painful (when done correctly with good positioning and a good latch). And when you become an expert breastfeeder, you don't even notice what it feels like!

When you get ready to pump for the first time, you may also be scared. Start at the lowest setting and work your way up. Again, it's going to feel like a tugging sensation, but it should not be painful. After pumping, your nipples will look weird and long, but they'll return to their normal shape within a few minutes. Use a double electric pump for the most efficiency, and don't forget to use LOTS of Lansinoh® cream on your nipples after breastfeeding and pumping to prevent cracking and discomfort. And use those breast pads when you use lanolin so you don't destroy your bras!

Two Babies and Two Breasts: There's No More Perfect Scenario

I firmly believe that having two babies and using both breasts for feeding them is a perfect and natural gift. Here are a few tips to enjoy this gift from the start:

✓ Do everything you can to get your babies to your breasts as soon as medically possible. Pump in the meantime.

✓ After giving birth, you will continue to feel contractions, especially while nursing. These contractions help your uterus to shrink back to its normal size, and breastfeeding your twins will make that happen faster.

✓ Be sure that your babies latch well. Your lactation consultant can help you with this. Your babies' bellies should be facing yours, and they should have your entire nipple and areola in their mouths.

BREASTFEEDING 3-DAY-OLD TWINS

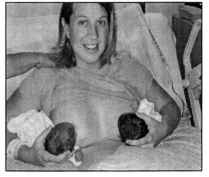

✓ As soon as you feel comfortable nursing one at a time, get both babies to both breasts to tandem breastfeed with the help of your lactation consultant. Try to tandem nurse from this point forward. As with anything, practice makes perfect. You can do this!

✓ Don't pull your babies off your nipples if you need to readjust them. Gently "break the seal" by inserting a finger into their mouths.

✓ Keep yourself healthy for your babies. To protect your back, bring your babies to your breasts instead of slouching over to bring your breasts to your babies. Accept help from others and delegate often...your only job is to breastfeed twins in the early days! Drink well, eat well, and get rest when you can. Also, keep stress to a minimum by having your spouse deal with family drama or trying situations.

Two Babies and Two Breasts: There's No More Perfect Scenario ...*But Things May Not Work Out Quite This Way!*

Lisa's Story
By Lisa Yarah, M.Ed., R.D., CD/N

My twins, Colden and Annaliese, were born three months prematurely and were in the NICU for nine weeks. I always planned on breastfeeding my twins exclusively, so I started pumping just a few hours after they were born. As a mother of twins in the NICU, I didn't really feel like a "mom" yet; so expressing breastmilk for my twins was the one thing I could do to feel connected to them. They received my breastmilk via a feeding tube until they were about 33 weeks gestational age.

Once they were developmentally ready to start nipple feeding, I worked closely with a lactation consultant who specialized in premature babies. Since premature babies have difficulty sucking, swallowing, and breathing all at the same time, she taught me how to look for their cues of distress. My son had particular difficulty latching on because his mouth was so small, so I had to use a nipple shield. We had to work closely with him, as he also experienced frequent hypoglycemia (low blood sugar). I became concerned he wasn't getting enough from my breast, so we had to supplement him with a bottle of my breastmilk after each breastfeeding session.

The lactation consultant worked with me on tandem feeding in preparation for home. Since the babies were hooked up to so many leads and monitors, I needed a lot of help from the nurses to tandem breastfeed. They also had frequent episodes of bradycardia (low heart rate) and apnea (period of not breathing) during their feedings, so I needed help pulling them off the breast quickly to pat them so that they would start breathing again. Since it would take about one to one and a half hours per nursing session, the nurses simply did not have the time to spend with me to feed them every three hours.

I started feeding them individually during the day every three hours, about an hour apart. At night, they received a bottle from the nurses. Since drinking breastmilk from the bottle required so much less energy expenditure and therefore less oxygen, they simply took to that better and could feed from a bottle in about 30 to 45 minutes per session.

When I got home, I tried to feed them exclusively from the breast. However, since they were hooked up to apnea monitors and still had frequent bradycardia and apnea events during the feedings, I found it nearly impossible to feed them by myself. I tried separating them by an hour, like in the NICU, but because it took so long per feeding and they were eating every two to three hours, I found myself glued to a chair all day long just breastfeeding. Even with my husband's support, I could not manage this on a day-to-day basis. I started just expressing my breastmilk for them and giving it to them in a bottle. The feedings then went quicker and smoother, and we were all a lot less stressed.

I felt extremely guilty over not physically breastfeeding, but I realized giving my breastmilk in the bottle was the next best thing and that my twins would still get just as much nutritional benefit from it if I planned their feedings wisely and used the freshest milk possible. I realized that I could still bond with them, even though they were not physically at my breast, just by sharing part of myself with them and knowing that I was doing what was best for them: giving them breastmilk.

Although my days were very busy with feeding the twins so often and then having to pump every three hours, I remained committed to giving them the very best I could offer. I found these tips imperative to my success:

1. **Invest in a good quality double pump.** You can pump both breasts at one time and therefore cut your pumping sessions in half.

2. **Enlist the support of your family.** Express your desire early on that you would like to provide your babies with the best start that nature has to offer, breastmilk, and this means that they will have to help out while you are expressing your breastmilk.

3. **Make the most of the time you spend pumping.** Since you are pumping so often, it is nice to actually get something accomplished while doing this. I hooked my pump up right at my desk and would write bills, work on the computer, etc., to use the time productively.

4. **Try to pump while the babies are sleeping.** I would do this and then make their bottles for their next feeding with the milk I just expressed; therefore, they would have the freshest milk possible and it would mimic actual, physical breastfeeding.

5. **If your babies are in the NICU, utilize the pumping room available at most NICUs.** I found it to be a great place to bond with other mothers and to share our stories while we were pumping. Be sure to bring water and a nutritious snack so that you can get nourishment while you pump. I would bring a cooler of water, fruit, yogurt and low-fat granola. I would get so hungry and thirsty while pumping, and having nutritious foods readily available made it easy to meet my increased energy needs when I was away from home.

6. **Purchase a car adaptor.** Since we were going to the NICU two to three times per day, I would spend my time in the car pumping while my husband was driving. This freed up time for me to do other things when I was home.

7. **Ask if you can use your friends'/neighbors'/family's freezers for storage.** You will not believe how much frozen breastmilk you will make,

and the NICU only lets you keep a certain amount in their freezer. Save every last drop, as you will need it all in the very near future!

8. **Last but not least, keep in mind what a wonderful thing you are doing for your babies, especially if they are premature.** There will be so many times when you will want to give up due to being so tired (especially when they come home from the NICU), but realize that this first year of life is so precious and that you will never get it back. It is relatively a short time period in one's life, and your self-sacrifice will benefit your twins *so much* in the future.

The benefits of breastfeeding preemies have been well documented. Research has shown that it is the perfect food, as it is higher in calories and protein than full-term milk, and it provides exactly what the premature infant needs in terms of immune factors. Breastfed preemies also experience greater weight gain and faster catch up growth. Breastmilk helps prevent infections, which are so common in the NICU and can be potentially deadly to a preemie (my kids never experienced any infections during their nine week stay in the NICU). Since preemies have immature digestive systems, they simply tolerate breastmilk better than formula and have less incidences of NEC (Necrotizing Enterocolitis), which is a serious inflammatory bowel disease. Most of all, breastfeeding is a wonderful way to bond with your babies when they are in the NICU. The closeness that you feel with them, even if you are solely pumping, helps you to truly feel like their "mother" before they come home from the hospital.

I fed my twins breastmilk solely for their first five months of life. At that time, they were eating more than I could pump, and I was running out of frozen breastmilk. Therefore, I had to start supplementing with bottles of formula in addition to the bottles of breastmilk I obtained from continued pumping. I still feel horribly guilty about providing supplemental formula, especially being a Registered Dietitian, but I know that I did the very best possible job that I could've done for my twins. Colden and Annaliese are almost caught up developmentally and physically (See "before" and "after" photos, next page), and I firmly believe that providing them with my breastmilk has helped them to grow and thrive as well as they have. I plan on continuing to pump until they are at least one year of age chronologically (their birthday), although I am hoping to make it to one year of age gestationally (their due date).

Lisa A. Yarah, M.Ed., R.D., CD/N is a mother of boy/girl twins, Colden and Annaliese (28 weekers) and is President of CNY Dietitian Consultants, Inc. Lisa can be reached via email at: lisard@twcny.rr.com.

"BEFORE" AND "AFTER" PHOTOS OF LISA'S TWINS

"Before:"
Colden Yarah
at birth, 2 lbs., 6 oz.

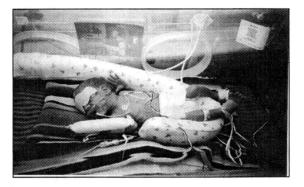

"Before:"
Annaliese Yarah
at birth, 2 lbs., 3 oz.

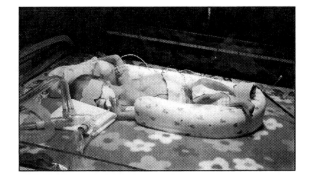

"After:" Colden and Annaliese at 5 ½ months old (Christmas 2006)

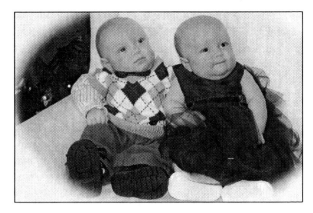

Chapter 17:
The First Days of Life with Twins

David and Julia left the hospital after a one-week stay in the NICU. Here are their stats upon leaving the hospital:

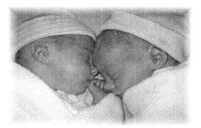

1 Week Old
David: 3 lbs., 14 oz.
Julia: 4 lbs., 2 ¾ oz.

My twins only stayed in the NICU for weight monitoring; and fortunately, they both took to breastfeeding fairly well. Both latched well, but we did have to work hard to reverse Julia's nipple confusion. Otherwise, breastfeeding had been getting easier...like learning to ride a bike!

The first days of life with twins at home were long, tired, challenging, special, and wonderful. In this timeframe, I developed my own system and became good at it, as you will too. As I mentioned, I dealt with nipple confusion and came up with my own solution. I also received constant support from my great lactation consultant, and she provided many tips along the way. In fact, I want to share some of my issues and some of my great lactation consultant's tips for success so that they may help you through some challenges:

✓ Before the babies come, get your breastfeeding contact information ready! This list should include your great lactation consultant's home phone and/or pager number and email address, a breastfeeding help line, a breastfeeding clinic number, and your local La Leche League phone number.

✓ Once you deliver your babies, be patient while learning to breastfeed twins! Both you and the babies have to learn this! And don't be afraid make your wishes known to the nursing staff.

✓ For nighttime feedings when only one baby awakens, **wake the other baby and tandem nurse so you can get your rest too.** Otherwise, if you nurse one baby at a time, you will end up being awake all night long feeding each baby individually!

✓ Wondering who gets which breast and when should you switch them? When it comes to confusion surrounding *assignment of breasts for each baby* versus *switching breasts at each feeding* versus *switching breasts mid-feeding*, go with what's simple! While tandem nursing, **give each baby his or her own breast for that feeding and then switch for the next feeding.** (It was at this point in time that I started my feeding log to keep this straight.) Or, some lactation consultants simply recommend assigning a breast to a baby for an entire day. (For me, this caused my breasts to become uneven since David suckled differently than Julia.) Do what works for you!

✓ Regarding your own tiredness and stress in those early days, remember: It's **okay** to take a night off and let your spouse give a bottle of BREASTMILK (bottles with orthodontic nipples). Just remember that you should pump for 15 minutes to make up for this missed feeding or else you will make less milk and become engorged! (Note: I never took the night off since I had incessant fears about my milk supply and making enough milk to support the growth of two babies!)

✓ Do not feed on a time schedule. Instead, **feed on demand for best success**; however, ask your doctor how much time can elapse before you should wake your babies to feed them. Usually in the beginning days, physicians will recommend feeding on demand but not going longer than three hours between feedings around the clock to promote optimal growth. Eventually, your doctor may allow the time between nighttime feeds to increase to every four hours before you should wake the babies.

✓ If your pumped quantity of milk starts to decrease around the one-month mark, know that your babies are becoming more efficient and are drinking more. Therefore, the quantity of milk that you pump after each feeding may be less than in the early days. Also, remember that your babies are ALWAYS more efficient than the pump! The babies may be getting far more milk than what you see in the pump containers.

✓ If you're wondering why your breasts become soft and flabby when your babies are about one month old, you are going through a "softening period" whereby engorgement stops.

✓ With increased demand (increased and/or longer feedings) comes increased milk supply. Every time you empty your breasts, you make milk at an even faster rate.

✓ When my first pediatrician told me not to let feedings last longer than 25 minutes since she felt that the breast "empties completely in 25 minutes," my lactation consultant told me not to put time limits on nursing. She told me that if the babies are demanding more, then give them more. This ensures a great milk supply, whereas time limits do just the opposite. And the breast never completely empties...it will continue making milk as long as your babies are suckling.

✓ Breastfeeding sessions may last anywhere from 15 minutes to 45 minutes. *However, don't watch the clock. Watch the babies for good positioning and a good latch.*

✓ When I was concerned that the babies were "taking" all of my milk at one feeding, leaving my breast feeling "empty" for the next feeding, my lactation consultant assured me that my breasts were still producing milk and adjusting to my babies' new nutritional needs.

✓ Take good care of your nipples:

   – Don't wash them with soap. Let water hit them in the shower to cleanse them. (NOTE: Before applying lanolin cream or a medicine cream for thrush, however, you can pat them with a warm washcloth.)

   – Get into the habit of squirting breastmilk onto your breasts after feedings as a natural "medicine" to prevent breast or nipple problems.

   – Also get into the habit of allowing your nipples to air dry. I did this by leaving my nursing bra "flaps" down underneath my shirt until they were dry. (And my husband would always say, "Hey! Your flaps are down!" since he could see through my shirt!)

   Many other issues arose during my babies' first six weeks of life. Since I had never before dealt with newborn babies, I had to do a lot of reading and researching for the littlest things. Here are a few of the things I learned:

Diapers

Based on the AAP (2004), your babies' diaper content should look like the following (See next page):

Urine
✓ As often as every 1 - 3 hours.

✓ Wet diapers at least 4 - 6 times a day.

✓ Could be light to darker yellow in color.

* Consult your pediatrician if your baby's urine is pinkish or if you find blood in the diaper.

Bowel Movements
✓ The first bowel movement is called meconium and is thick, dark green, or black.

✓ Once meconium is passed, stool turns yellowish-green.

✓ Then stools will turn soft or runny, mustard-colored, and seedy if your babies are solely breastfed. The stools will look like this until you add solids, which then make their poop look like a softer and mushier version of ours!

✓ Normal stooling varies from baby to baby. Breastfed babies may poop after every feeding; or by three to six weeks of age, they may only poop once or twice a week and not be considered constipated as long as poop is still soft. This is because breastmilk clears the bowels almost entirely. If your babies are otherwise gaining weight steadily, nursing well, and have soft poop, there shouldn't be any issues with a decrease in stooling. But as always, consult your doctor if you are worried.

✓ If stools ever look hard or very dry, your baby may not be getting enough fluids.

✓ Stools can be any color of the rainbow; however, consult your pediatrician if stools contain blood, mucus, or water.

* For more exact information on diaper content for brand new newborns, see Chapter 8, Breasts A & P.

Hunger Signals

Breastfeed promptly and on demand when you notice the following hunger signals:

✓ Restless sleep, squirminess, or increased alertness.

✓ Smacking lips or mouthing.

✓ Rooting or mouth opening in search of the nipple. (Rooting can occur when you stroke the babies' cheeks with your finger or nipple.)

✓ Becoming fussy.

✓ Remember, crying is a late hunger signal, and a crying baby at the breast takes in more air which leads to GAS (which leads to more crying)!

✓ In the early days, your babies may want to breastfeed as often as every hour or hour and a half. This is only temporary...so let them!

Signs That Your Babies Are Not Thriving

Rosenthal & Arsenault (2001) list several signs that indicate that your babies may not be thriving. If you notice any of these signs, notify your pediatrician immediately:

✓ Less than 6 soaked diapers in 24 hours.

✓ Persistent diarrhea.

✓ Persistent and worsening jaundice or yellowing of the skin.

✓ Fever. (Can indicate infection or illness – ask your pediatrician what temperature they consider a fever.)

✓ Persistent weight loss.

✓ Persistent crying that does not let up.

Supplemental Nutrition and Pumping

Many premature babies need supplemental nutrition in order to gain weight more quickly. If you have premature babies who need supplemental nutrition, the supplemental bottle should follow each breastfeeding and should consist of breastmilk or breastmilk fortified with human milk fortifier/premature baby formula powder in a specific quantity to make your milk higher in calories. Consult your doctor or dietitian before you add anything to your breastmilk and ask what quantity is appropriate. There are very specific mathematical formulas to determine a calorie level for your babies' supplements.

In my case, I gave fortified 30 cc supplemental bottles after every feeding from birth until my twins reached six pounds, which happened to be the six-week mark. At six pounds, my pediatrician then recommended weaning them off the bottles slowly by reducing supplemental bottles to every other feed for one week. After that week, we ended supplemental bottles! Hooray! However, I was so afraid that my babies would not continue to grow at the same rate... I am happy to report that they very successfully became normal, thriving, solely breastfed babies!

Be sure to ask your doctor how long you will need to give supplemental bottles of breastmilk and for recommendations for weaning off these bottles. Also ask if he or she recommends a vitamin supplement and which one would be appropriate. At six weeks, my babies began a vitamin supplement with iron and Vitamin D (which are in very low quantities in breastmilk). Some vitamins can be purchased over the counter and others are only available by a prescription. Your pediatrician will let you know which one to purchase. But heed this warning: VITAMINS WITH IRON TASTE GROSS AND BABIES MAY GAG ON THEM. Therefore, be sure to use bibs when giving vitamins!

I let my twins gag the vitamins down as best they could, and some was always spit out. The good news is that once your babies start on iron-fortified cereals at four to six months, the vitamin may change to an iron-free, fluoride vitamin, which tastes MUCH better! (Fluoride is recommended in areas where water is not fluoridated – See Appendix C.)

As I mentioned earlier, I pumped my breasts after every single feeding around the clock from day one to obtain extra breastmilk for all the supplemental bottles and to ensure that I had a great milk supply. At six weeks, however, we no longer needed supplemental bottles. Therefore, my pediatrician recommended pumping after every other feeding to keep my milk supply up and to continue to have a supply of breastmilk in the freezer.

By eight weeks, my pediatrician recommended pumping only when I wanted. This scared me since I already had constant anxiety about my milk supply; however, letting my now more efficient babies feed on demand worked remarkably well in keeping my milk supply just where it needed to be!

Pacifiers

Don't use them quite yet...wait until your babies are older than six to eight weeks to prevent nipple confusion and to ensure successful breastfeeding. See the next chapter for more information on paci's.

Awakening a Sleepy Baby at the Breast

A very common problem with nursing tiny, premature babies is keeping them awake enough to breastfeed. I found the following strategies helpful:

✓   Rub their heads.

✓   Stroke their feet.

✓   Rub their cheeks (which can trigger the rooting reflex, making baby want to suckle).

✓   Rub their backs.

✓   Pick them up and talk to them.

✓   Rub a cool washcloth on their face, arms, or legs.

✓   Change their diapers.

✓   Undress them.

✓   Sing to them.

✓   Tickle them (as a last resort).

Clothing for Tiny Babies

In department stores, you may find a full premature baby clothing section with lots of cute items. My babies were born in the summer, so family went crazy purchasing little shorts outfits, dresses, bathing suits, sleeveless rompers, etc.

However, my babies were born at low birth weights with temperature regulation problems and needed to keep warm since they didn't have enough brown fat, or the type of fat that acts as insulation. Therefore, the most practical outfits for your twins' first weeks of life are warm sleepers with feet. I also used socks under these. In fact, for the first two weeks of their lives, they wore these sleepers along with a tight swaddle consisting of two receiving blankets to keep them warm!

It was not until my babies were three or four weeks old that I started using some of those cute preemie clothes that were more seasonal. I did, however, continue to use warm sleepers for nighttime. In fact, I put footed sleepers on my twins for nighttime for the whole first year! I used fleecy or terry styles in the cold months, and I switched to thinner, cotton versions for the warmer months. And I never had a need to use the blanket sleepers since my babies were warm enough with their pajamas alone. I feared that these seemingly practical devices would overheat my children, which is a Sudden Infant Death Syndrome (SIDS) risk. Just make sure your room temperature is not too cool or too warm, for that matter. You should feel comfortable in the babies' room in just a t-shirt, and they should always wear one more layer than you.

Bathing Your Twins

You cannot bathe your babies in a tub of water until their umbilical stump falls off and until the penis is completely healed from the circumcision for boys. Your pediatrician will alert you as to when bathing in a tub is appropriate. Up until that point, use a bucket or hospital basin filled with water and mild soap for sponge baths.

When you can finally give that first bath, I recommend using a hospital basin or an adjustable baby tub with suction cups with an adult-sized washcloth covering the bottom to prevent slipping. Tiny babies are very slippery, especially in the hands of inexperienced parents! As your babies grow, you can bathe them one at a time in an infant tub placed inside your bathtub, which makes cleanup less time consuming. And you can bathe them one at a time in this tub until they are great at sitting up (eight months or beyond). Then, you can put them in the regular bathtub with an anti-skid mat. (Babies remain slippery little people for a long time!)

When your babies are good at sitting up unassisted and you are feeling confident, you can try bathing them together to save time. I started this at eight months with my husband as my helper. We each washed a baby and it worked out very well! You can try to bathe your babies alone at this time as well, but know that once they start standing up in the tub, you should go back to bathing them with a helper to prevent falls.

As far as how often you should bathe your babies, aim for a good bath every other day and a sponge bath in between with water or mildly soapy water and a washcloth. (Avoid extra soap in the winter as it can cause dry skin.) You can continue this routine until the babies start running around and getting really dirty (or if they like to smear their food in their hair and ears regularly!).

Sleeping and Napping

Newborn premature twins sleep a lot. In fact, they sleep a lot until they are four or five months old! Other mom friends of mine talked about how their four month olds had a nap schedule, but my babies had much the same sleep routine as when they were newborns: Wake up in the morning, nurse, sleep. Wake up, nurse, sleep. Wake up, nurse, play for a little while, sleep. Wake up, nurse, read books, sleep. And so on until bedtime. At five months old, however, a routine emerged where my babies woke up, nursed, remained awake for a while, and then napped. They had two to three naps a day at this time, which stuck until they were over a year old.

As far as *where* to sleep, I put my babies in the same room to promote bonding and a safe, secure emotional environment. In my opinion, this helped their health and growth, and I do hope they will have a strong relationship for years to come. And always, always, always put your babies on their **backs** to sleep!

Some moms feel safer with their babies in their room; however, I believe that babies need to learn to sleep in their own space. And they are not alone in their room; they have each other. Just use a baby monitor and be sure the nursery in your home is not too far from your room so that you can attend to them as needed.

Vaccinations

As for vaccination appointments, remember that you as a mother will have to endure the amount of vaccines times two. Here are two helpful hints:

✓ You will absolutely need a helper for vaccination doctor's appointments! Never try it alone...not until your twins can walk! Even then, I still recommend a team of two for these appointments since your children will both need to be comforted!

✓ In the beginning, I was worried about my own breastfeeding modesty and tried to give my crying twins bottles of breastmilk after their shots. Since they never otherwise got bottles, this was traumatizing! They not only got stuck with needles, but then they got a hard plastic nipple and a cold bottle of breastmilk! At their three-month appointment, I finally came to the realization that I was making these appointments worse by giving my babies bottles. I brought in my breastfeeding pillow and wore a shirt conducive to modest breastfeeding, and then I nursed my upset babies immediately after their shots! They not only got yummy and warm breastmilk, but they also got the comfort of Mommy! My advice to you is to do this from the start! The nurses in pediatrician's offices will support this too!

Growth Spurts

Growth or "appetite" spurts occur around specific times, and they come on strong, especially if your babies were premature and need to catch up on growth. Major growth spurts can be expected around the following times according to AAP (2004):

✓ 8-12 days old.
✓ 3-4 weeks.
✓ 6 weeks.
✓ 3 months.
✓ Other times as well, especially if your babies are premature.

Growth spurts can be demanding on your time and energy since breastfeeding will increase dramatically in frequency and in duration. At six weeks, I remember feeling like all I did was nurse my babies and get a few moments of rest in between. My twins were just constantly hungry, and I remember nursing them every hour or so for 30 to 45 minutes total! I was a human milk machine! I thought I would go crazy, but this only ended up lasting two or three days. And after this happened the first time, I researched growth spurts and knew when to expect the next one. Luckily, by three and a half months old, I found that marathon breastfeeding due to growth spurts had ceased forever!

Reflux

Gastroesophageal reflux in babies is common, and most babies will outgrow it before their first birthday. In my case, David had started doing some strange things during and after feedings. He'd whimper at feedings, turn pale, suckle less at the breast, arch his back, act lethargic, and spit up excessively. I became very worried and feared weight loss, so I called the pediatrician immediately. We went to the doctor, and he said that David probably had reflux. Our doctor also told us about prescribing Zantac®, but he wanted to wait to see if the symptoms persisted.

Then one night, my husband, my sister, and I were watching TV while I was breastfeeding David and Julia. All of a sudden, David choked on some breastmilk. I picked him up quickly and noticed that he couldn't breathe. He started to turn blue or cyanotic, and my husband grabbed him from me, turned him upside down facing the floor, and started burping him forcefully. We heard a huge gasp of air, and then David's normal color returned. We immediately called the emergency pediatrician phone number, and the physician on-call said that this was probably classic reflux.

The next day, David went for a barium swallow, and sure enough he had reflux. He was prescribed Zantac® immediately and did great from that point forward. One thing to remember with anti-reflux medications, however, is to remind your physician that your baby is growing and needs an increase in the dose. Our pediatric office was very busy, and appointments were therefore very brief. I had to proactively ask the doctor if David needed more medicine as he was growing because I noticed that symptoms were returning on the initial prescribed dose.

For babies, some spitting up is normal, but gastroesophageal reflux is not. Some symptoms of reflux include frequent and severe spitting up, forceful vomiting; back arching; not taking the breast when offered; grunting or crying after nursing; swallowing difficulty including gagging or choking; and frequent hiccupping or burping (The National Women's Health Information Center, 2006). If you suspect that one or both of your babies has reflux, mention it to your pediatrician. If your baby has reflux and turns blue, lethargic, and/or stops breathing, immediately have someone call 911 and immediately attempt to burp your baby, face down. If the baby returns to his normal state, call your pediatric office regardless to see what you should do next.

To alleviate symptoms of reflux in your breastfed baby, you can keep your baby's head higher than her feet during feedings by using a footstool or two nursing pillows around your waist. Keep your baby upright after feedings as well. If your baby is on reflux medications, do not skip doses and be sure to give the medicine at the same times daily. To prevent choking, it also helps to keep your baby awake during feedings (See suggestions mentioned earlier in this chapter).

Colic (Or Babies that have a "Fussy Time")

Although Julia had stopped crying at the breast because of nipple confusion, she began crying everyday at 4:00 pm and cried in between her naps for the rest of the evening until bedtime. I swore she had colic, which includes incessant crying later in the day, pulling of legs and passing gas, and sensitivity to stimulation. In essence, Julia's "fussy time" or colic lasted from about six weeks to three months old, which is consistent with colic. It was funny...Julia's "fussy time" was always during dinner time, so my husband and I got used to eating dinner with Julia's crying as our background music!

Here are some ways to ease colic or crying during a "fussy time:"

✓ Ask your pediatrician when you can safely use a baby swing. I introduced Julia to her swing at six weeks old and used it twice a day for no more than a half an hour at each session as a colic cure for her!

✓ Use an exercise ball and *gently* bounce on the ball with your baby in your lap. (Don't shake your baby! If you ever feel as though you want to shake or harm your baby, seek help from your doctor or from a licensed professional counselor.)

✓ Try a vibrating infant chair.

✓ Rock him or walk with him.

✓ Nurse her...she may be hungry!

✓ Get her away from stimulation. Excessive noise, light, or other stimuli may be bothering her.

✓ On the other hand, sometimes singing softly or playing soft music will make him calm.

✓ This sounds weird, but take her outside. Perhaps your home is feeling stuffy or your air temperature is not comfortable for your baby. If your home is too cool or warm, adjust your thermostat. (A great tip for temperature control is that your baby should have one more layer on than you, and you should feel comfortable in your home in a t-shirt.) With Julia, we learned that she didn't like the air conditioning too cool because she stopped crying when we took her outside in the warm summer sun!

✓ Swaddle him.

✓ Put her on her belly to help her pass gas.

✓ Ask your pediatrician about using gas drops.

✓ Think about what you've eaten...has something you've eaten made you gassy? This could've also made baby gassy. Make a list of all the foods that do this and avoid them until your babies are four to six months old.

✓ I have to mention this suggestion, but with some rules: You can use a pacifier, as your baby may need to fulfill sucking needs; however, **wait until they are older than six weeks** or else you may cause severe breastfeeding problems or nipple confusion! (There's more on this in the next chapter.)

Tummy Time

At four weeks old, my pediatrician also suggested that the babies start some "tummy time." Since babies should ALWAYS be put on their backs to sleep to reduce the risk of SIDS, they begin to need some time on their stomachs for large muscle development while awake during the day. Tummy time also gives them some time on the floor with you for interaction. To start, put your babies on the floor on a soft, thin blanket. Place them on their tummies with their heads to the side until they no longer wish to be in this position. You'll know they want to go back to their backs when they appear frustrated or start to cry.

Last, But Not Least: Breastfeeding "Brand New" Newborns

Breastfeeding brand new newborns may include 8 to 12 (or more!) feedings per day, and feedings may last anywhere from 15 to 45 minutes (or more!). Follow your babies' leads, and don't set limits on the number of feedings per day or the amount of time each feeding should last. Feed on demand for best success, and know that all this nursing is only temporary.

To Sum Up

To sum up, I want to share with you the top 10 things I learned during the early days of life with twins:

1. I learned that it's okay to go to bed at 9:00 pm when you need to get up every three hours throughout the entire night. In fact, I learned that this was the smartest and healthiest decision I could ever have made!

2. Along the same lines, I learned that it's okay to "sleep in" around feedings until 11:00 am to catch up on needed rest.

3. I learned that you, the parent, ultimately set the babies' routine based on your behaviors. You CAN get your babies to think it is "nighttime" until 11:00 am to get them to sleep in as well.

4. I learned that twins are two very different human beings with different needs, habits, preferences, and personalities.

5. Along these lines, I learned that twins don't always sleep at the same time. The old saying, "Sleep when your baby sleeps" doesn't apply with twins.

6. I learned that if you keep consistent with a routine, your babies feel safe and secure and will know what to expect. They WILL come to know that they should sleep through the night and take naps at the same time...I promise! Be consistent.

7. Pre-pregnancy, I felt tired when I got seven hours of uninterrupted sleep. I always needed at least eight hours of sleep each night. I now know that I NEVER knew what tired was back then!

8. I learned that all difficult things are temporary and only make you a stronger human being. If you keep trying your hardest, you'll eventually get through difficult times and succeed in the process.

9. I learned that breastfeeding is amazing and remarkable in terms of helping you and your babies bond, helping your babies to grow more quickly (from the superior nutritional quality and from being close to Mommy's skin), and acting as a protective medicine for your immune-suppressed tiny babies.

10. I learned that breastfeeding twins is a full-time job with overtime hours. I also learned that breastfeeding twins is the best, most rewarding job I've ever had!

Chapter 18:
Six Weeks to Four Months Old

Other than spending most of my days topless, nothing too eventful happened from the six week to four-month timeframe. Here are the babies' stats:

	6 weeks old	4 months old
David:	5 lbs. 15 oz., 20 in.	11 lbs. 8 oz., 25 in.
Julia:	6 lbs. 8 oz., 20 in.	11 lbs. 10 oz., 24 in.

We got over nipple confusion by six weeks, and David was diagnosed with reflux and being treated effectively with Zantac®. In addition, I swore Julia had colic, but I'll just call it a "fussy time," which did eventually resolve around four months old. And then growth spurts hit at three weeks and six weeks old, but we got through those too. But at two and a half months old, the growth spurts and increased cries for the breast combined with Julia's "fussy time" crying led me to a breaking point: Using the dreaded pacifier!

Pacifiers

I am definitely an anti-pacifier person. I don't like looking at big toddlers with "binkies," and I never wanted to get my kids into such a bad habit. But the frequent need to suck along with what I will call Julia's "fussy time" forced me to look into other options. I went through mental agony regarding using pacifiers, and I even called my great lactation consultant to ask for her input. She told me that moms should definitely wait until their babies are older than six weeks to introduce a pacifier so as not to cause nipple confusion and breastfeeding problems, but that it is a medical fact that babies need to suck. And with twins, a breastfeeding mom can easily become a human pacifier to fulfill two babies' sucking needs.

I gave my babies pacifiers. David hated the paci, and he always spit it out. (I kept offering the pacifier to him when I would give one to Julia to be fair, but he preferred his thumb.) Julia, on the other hand, loved the paci (initially), which changed her disposition dramatically! Who knew that something as simple as using a pacifier would make my "fussy" child stop crying! All she wanted was some extra sucking, and she found her thumb soon after as well which caused her to lose interest in the pacifier.

By four months, neither one of my babies had a desire for a pacifier. I threw them away (okay, I hid them in the back of a drawer…just in case) and would never have to deal with weaning a big, walking, and talking toddler from the pacifier.

Consider the following about pacifiers:

1. If you NEED to introduce a pacifier for your babies' sucking needs (and to resign from your job as human pacifier), wait as long as possible so as not to cause problems with breastfeeding. **Wait until your babies are six weeks or older.**

2. If they don't take to it, don't push it! And if they prefer their thumbs, that's okay too.

3. If at any point in time they seem to lose interest and are over their sucking needs or fussy moods, ditch the pacifiers! It's easier to get a little infant off a pacifier than a toddler who uses their pacifier as a comfort item or "lovey!" Habits are easier to break when they are newer habits and when your babies are younger.

Strange Breastfeeding Occurrences

Between six weeks and four months old, I did experience some strange breastfeeding-related occurrences. Read on for my weird stories!

Cabbage: Not the Best Menu Choice for Me
When the babies were 10 weeks old, I celebrated my 27th birthday at a Japanese hibachi grill, my favorite type of restaurant. While I knew I would have to forego the raw sushi, I did enjoy the hibachi grilled chicken, rice, and vegetables, which included cabbage. While breastfeeding, I had always feared even touching cabbage because I had heard about its reputation as being something that can "dry up your milk." (If you have a plugged duct, you can put a cabbage leaf on your breast to pull out the clogged milk. Overusing this technique, however, can dry up your milk.) I also knew that cabbage makes many people gassy, but is was my birthday! I ate the cabbage!

Well, the cabbage did make me gassy. Other breastfeeding moms had warned me about limiting or avoiding gassy foods during breastfeeding to prevent giving the babies gas. I knew this, but that food smelled so good! I truly enjoyed it…and the next day, Julia had blood in her diaper.

I frantically called the pediatrician's office, and they asked me to come in immediately with Julia *and* the diaper. After examining the diaper, the physician asked me a simple question, "What did you eat yesterday?" I simply replied, "Cabbage." Well, it turned out that Julia had gotten such bad gas from the soy-saucy, cabbage-flavored breastmilk that she needed to strain to release the gas, causing a small tear in her rectum! My advice: be cautious or even avoid the foods that give you major gas, as these can also give your babies major gas! Needless to say, my pediatrician informed me that rectal tears are rarely serious and heal on their own without the need for medications or creams.

A Strange Itchy Sensation
Another rather unpleasant thing happened in this timeframe as well. I had been a faithful user of Lansinoh® cream. When I saw any cracking or dryness on my nipples, I gooped it on generously. Problem solved. However, it was late August, and my nipples became very sore. I thought that maybe I had been sweaty from the heat, causing my nipples to become infected or cracked from sweat. Breastfeeding had never before hurt me. I knew it wasn't supposed to hurt, but it became unbearable. I pulled out all my favorite breastfeeding books to look up what ailment I could have, but my pain didn't match any of the descriptions. My nipples were so painful that I didn't know how much longer I could take it. I never used so much nipple cream in my life!

Then I remembered something: Two weeks prior, I noticed a white spot on Julia's tongue. It had to be thrush! At our next pediatric visit, I pointed it out. The physician said, "It's not thrush. Thrush starts on the cheek." Well, always trust your instincts...it *was* thrush. And when left untreated, your other baby can get thrush too from *your* breasts! Then, all three of you will be in pain. My babies continued to suckle fine, but some babies stop suckling since the pain is so severe. Be a proactive patient and ask for thrush medicine immediately. You'll regret it otherwise.

What ended up happening was that Julia gave it to me, and I gave it to David. Julia got better, but then she got re-infected from my breasts. And because none of us were treated, the thrush or yeast on my nipples kept growing and producing even more pain. There was literally a fungus among us, and we needed treatment! Once we all got some Nystatin, we were on our way to recovery! But this was, by far, the most painful breastfeeding ailment of all!

If you notice white spots *anywhere* in your babies' mouths, tell the pediatrician immediately and get everyone treated or you will have to endure this horrible pain! Doctors may also write one prescription for you to "share" with the babies. Don't do this! Ask your doctor for your own prescription (which is usually the same prescription that the babies have). Otherwise, none of you will get enough medicine to kill this fungus quickly and effectively! (See Chapter 9 for more information on breast pain and thrush.)

I had a few other experiences within the six week to four month timeframe that could have been easier or less stressful had I received tips from other moms first. Read on so you won't have to endure the same level of stress!

Don't Take Any Medication Without Asking a Doctor First

In this time frame, I also discovered that simple medications that I commonly took without even thinking prior to my pregnancy/lactation days now could cause HUGE problems for breastfeeding babies! In my case, I was having some diarrhea and decided to take some anti-diarrheal medication. Well, after I took the tablets, I thought, "Oh NO!" I immediately called the pediatrician's office, and they said that my breastmilk for the next two feedings would definitely cause severe constipation for my babies. Their recommendation: Feed the babies bottles of breastmilk from the freezer instead. And at the times when my babies were due to feed, I had to pump and dump my "constipation-causing" milk. The moral of the story is: Ask your pediatrician or physician what medications are safe and in what quantity you may use them while you are lactating.

Puke

I also need to mention puke: Some babies spit up more than others; however, my son was (and still is) a major puker. Even on Zantac®, David still spit up occasionally. Therefore, I will recommend that you always be prepared with something to wipe spit-up if your babies tend to be pukers. And if you are dressed nicely, use a burp rag or have a spare outfit ready. If you hand your baby who is a puker to an innocent bystander, give them a burp rag or else you will need to give them a Shout wipe (which is a diaper bag necessity with pukers) or money towards their dry cleaning! Also, know that if your babies are pukers, the spit up gets really stinky when you start solids. Please ask your doctor about your babies' spitting up if you feel it is excessive or if you feel that your babies may have reflux.

Hair and Nails

Somewhere between two and four months, you and your babies will start losing your hair. You will notice more hair in your shower drain and comb, and the babies will either go completely bald or have that "thinning, receding hairline" look. By around six months, however, your hair should stop falling out and the babies should be getting some hair. Although, it is normal for a baby to be completely bald for their first year of life!

I mention this so that you don't think that either you or your babies are malnourished. It is completely normal for both you and your babies to lose hair due to hormonal changes. If you or your babies have other accompanying symptoms, you can certainly ask your physician about hair loss to be safe.

As for nails, this is a warning: Get comfortable trimming your babies' fingernails quickly and often! And get some good safety baby clippers. You will need to trim 20 baby fingernails every three days or so! You can do this successfully either while the babies are sleeping to prevent squirming or on the changing table for stability when they are little (when they are toddlers: good luck to you!). Luckily, baby toenails don't grow as quickly. Your nails will also grow more quickly due to your prenatal vitamins.

To trim the babies' fingernails, cut them straight across the middle first, and then cut each side to get rid of sharp edges and round off the nail. To trim toenails, trim them straight across the middle only. You can also trim sharp edges as needed. In my case, it helped to sing a song to get the babies to relax while trimming nails (if they were not asleep during nail cutting sessions).

Carpal Tunnel Symptoms

By holding two babies' heads in my hands while nursing eight to ten times a day for 20 to 45 minutes at a time, I began experiencing carpal tunnel symptoms in both hands around the three month mark, and these strange symptoms recurred on occasion in the later months of my breastfeeding career. More specifically, I experienced this numbness in my hands mainly at night. The numbness would actually wake me up. If you experience this same sensation in your hands and it becomes painful, talk to your doctor, as you may have carpal tunnel syndrome!

Trips to the Store

An interesting thing will happen when you take your adorable twin babies to the store or anywhere else in public: EVERYONE WILL STOP TO LOOK AT, TOUCH, OR TALK TO YOUR BABIES. And then they will proceed to talk to you and ask you a hundred questions about your babies. If you are in a long checkout line, this does come in handy to pass the time. But otherwise, it gets old very quickly. Don't get me wrong...all this attention is flattering. And when you run out on a quick errand by yourself, you may feel unimportant and unnoticed without your babies. But if you're out with your babies and you've nursed them before leaving the house, knowing they will need to eat again in approximately 80 minutes, and you have a long grocery list, people stopping you becomes really annoying! For the first five to 10 times this happens, enjoy it. It's flattering. After that, ignore people. Keep walking. Answer their questions with one-word answers and a nice smile, and then proceed with your shopping. Otherwise, you're going to have some really unhappy babies who want your breastmilk NOW! Then you will need to either breastfeed on a hard bench (which can be uncomfortable and distracting depending on the location) or breastfeed in the car. Home is definitely the most comfortable place to nurse your babies. See Chapter 13 for more tips on breastfeeding while out or while traveling.

As for touching your babies, you need to do everything possible to keep your babies healthy. For example, if you're babies' health is still shaky, don't take them out yet. If it's the middle of winter and cold season, limit your trips out as well. If you know that a family member has a cold and will be hosting a party, it's okay not to attend the party. If people in Wal-Mart® blatantly reach over to touch your baby, you can either ask that they not touch your premature baby or pull out the baby wipes to wipe off the germs once the person has left. Or, to make a lasting effect on the person, pull out the baby wipes and wipe off the germs right then and there!

"Neh Pachai Hovenko Ked Neh Smedzie!"

Please excuse my spelling if you know Slovak (and please pardon me if there are curse words in this phrase), but this is a saying that my Slovak grandmother taught me, which I want to share with you. "Don't sniff the poop if it doesn't stink!" What this means, in simple terms, is don't bother peaceful babies. If they happen to fall asleep on the floor and you'd prefer them to sleep in their cribs, don't go and move them. You'll wake them up and have unhappy and crabby babies to contend with. If your babies are playing by themselves in their cribs while you catch up on some dishes, don't disturb them. Basically, in any scenario, don't disturb a peaceful baby unless safety becomes an issue. Otherwise, as long as they are safe, leave peaceful babies alone!

Listen to Other People's Advice with a Cautious Ear

Yes, listen to trusted health professionals and physicians' advice (remembering that even these folks are human and can be wrong, in which case a second opinion is a great option), but be weary of random advice from family, friends, or strangers.

For example:

✓ My mom, a formula mom, told me that I should give the babies a bottle once in a while so they would take it in my absence. In asking my pediatrician about this, however, I learned that hungry babies would suckle to obtain milk...even from a bottle in dire situations.

✓ Grandma told me that I would not be able to feed my babies when they hit 12 lbs. because they would be too squirmy. When they were 12 lbs., they were a joy to feed. Then she said, "You won't be able to feed them at 15 lbs." Well, yes they were inclined to squirm more at 15 lbs. But when it was time to eat, it was business only for my babies. They nursed just fine. And as big, walking toddlers, they still nursed great!

✓ Grandma also told me that my milk must be "of poor quality" when the babies were six weeks old because they were nursing every hour and a half. When I asked my pediatrician about this, she said that my milk was "of the finest vintage" since my babies were gaining two pounds per month, every month. Truth is, the reason my babies were nursing so much is that they were hitting a growth spurt, needing additional "catch up" growth, and developing non-nutritive sucking needs!

✓ Too many people told me that I would either not be able to nurse twins past six weeks or that I would eventually need to supplement with formula. Or they would tell me about "a friend" who failed in attempting to breastfeed her multiples. What do I have to say to them now? "OH YES YOU CAN BREASTFEED TWINS!" I successfully breastfed my two babies for two years!

RSV Vaccinations

One last thing that I need to mention is that premature babies are at higher risk for developing respiratory syncytial virus (RSV), which can impact lung function, cause hospitalization, or even death. There is a vaccination to protect your premature babies, so be sure to ask your physician about having your babies vaccinated. Usually you need to contact your insurance provider as well to be sure they will cover this very costly vaccination. This vaccination is typically administered to premature or at-risk babies every month from October through April. Once your babies hit the 15 lb. mark, the dose typically increases to an additional shot.

Last, But Not Least: Breastfeeding Six Week to Four Month Olds

Breastfeeding six week to four month olds will require a lot of energy and time. They're hungry little guys and will go through several growth spurts in this timeframe. Breastfeeding will include 8 to 10 (or more!) feedings per day, and feedings may last anywhere from 15 to 45 minutes (or more!). Follow your babies' leads, and don't set limits on the number of feedings per day or the amount of time each feeding should last. Feed on demand for best success, and know that all this nursing is only temporary. After four months, nursing does slow down a bit, and the amount of time at your breasts should lessen a bit too.

To Sum Up

To sum up, I want to share with you the top 10 things I learned during the six week to four month old timeframe:

1. Sometimes you don't realize how hard something was until after you've been through it. You just do what you need to do when it needs to be done. Then, you can look back on the difficult time with a sense of inner strength and say, "It's so much easier now, and I'm such a strong and resilient person!"

2. With double the babies, you need to be double the planner and organizer.

3. Just when you think you've figured out your babies, they change. Accept that the only constant thing is change!

4. During this timeframe, you will need to accept the fact that your main job in life is to breastfeed two babies. In accepting this fact, you will have a true focus and you will be a success.

5. In addition, you will need to accept the fact that you cannot be everything for everyone. Your number one priority is to feed your babies and get them to grow. Laundry, housework, returned phone calls to friends, etc. will just have to wait, and that is okay.

6. Along the same lines, your babies come first. Sometimes you just may need to hurt others' feelings to protect your babies. This is okay too. If they truly love you, they'll get over it.

7. With little tiny twins, there are just some things you are not going to be able to do alone. You'll need a helper at times. Ask for and accept help to make things more feasible.

8. By four months, you can truly say to yourself, "I'm really good at this, and I deserve a lot of credit."

9. By four months, you can also say, "Where has the time gone?" It truly does fly...enjoy every moment with your precious little miracles!

10. Prior to having babies, you could never even imagine how much your heart would burst with love for these tiny perfect people!

Chapter 19:
Five to Seven Months Old

At five months old, you may discover that something has changed without you even realizing it was happening. Could all this be getting easier? At the same time, your babies become more alert, more independent, and more skilled with their bodies, which can create new difficulties for you. At this time, there is a lot of change for the better, but some of this change comes with a price tag attached. First, my babies' stats:

	5 months old	7 months old
David:	12 lbs. 12 oz., 25 ½ in.	15 lbs. 0 oz.
Julia:	12 lbs. 12 oz., 24 in.	15 lbs. 5 oz.

Sleeping through the Night

Oh, the first time the babies sleep through the night is magical! You will discover that you never knew what good sleep was until that first full week of sleeping through the night. It's truly great! And after the babies have been sleeping through the night for a month or so, you might think, "How did I survive on so little sleep?"

There is one thing, however, that other breastfeeding moms may forget to tell you regarding your babies sleeping through the night: PAIN! I didn't know about this; no one warned me. I want to warn you: As your babies begin sleeping for longer stretches through the night, you will begin to become engorged again. You actually become engorged to the same degree that you were engorged when your milk first came in. It feels like your breasts are going to pop! They won't though, I promise! Anyway, your babies start sleeping for longer stretches, but your body is still programmed to produce milk every so many hours. Basically, your body needs to adjust to the decreased need for milk overnight, causing your breasts to be extremely engorged until your body "gets it."

My babies started off by sleeping from 9:00 pm until 3:30 am. This caused severe engorgement, which lasted for about four nights. Then, my body adjusted and the pain lessened slightly. Then, the babies started sleeping from 9:00 pm until 5:30 am, which was wonderful and painful at the same time. This engorgement, on the other hand, was so extremely painful that I pumped for 10 minutes to relieve the pain. This was counterproductive in that I was "telling" my body to make milk at a time of day when I needed to "train" my body to stop making so much milk (at night). The pain was severe, and it felt like my nipples were burning. I thought I'd pop! But in time, the pain passed and my body adjusted.

Don't give in to pumping...it will just prolong things. (If in terrible pain, pump off five minutes of milk.) Eventually, my babies began sleeping from 9:00 pm to 9:00 am (See Chapter 3 on creating a bedtime ritual), which was great. And eventually I stopped becoming terribly engorged. But I'll warn you about one more thing: I never stopped leaking overnight and needed breast pads for leakage overnight for the first eight to nine months. In the later months, during some nights, I never leaked a drop. Other nights, however, my leaking milk quantity ranged from drips to buckets. Get some good overnight breast pads and use them faithfully for a majority of your lactating days (and nights!).

Another good thing to know is that formula-fed babies start sleeping through the night sooner than breastfed babies...A LOT SOONER! Perhaps they may start at six or eight weeks old! PLEASE DON'T USE FORMULA TO GET YOUR BABIES TO SLEEP THROUGH THE NIGHT! The reason that formula-fed babies sleep through the night sooner is because a pile of sludge (otherwise known as formula) is sitting in their immature digestive tracts. This milk-based sludge (You know that babies aren't supposed to start milk until one year old, right?) is so difficult to digest that it gives a feeling of fullness, which therefore allows the baby to sleep for longer periods of time. A breastfed baby, on the other hand, clears almost his entire digestive tract when he poops since breastmilk leaves behind very little waste after a bowel movement. This is also why your babies will poop more than formula-fed babies...it's called quick transit time. This is also why formula-fed babies are often constipated to the degree of severe discomfort.

It's funny: When I asked my pediatrician at around four months when my babies would start sleeping through the night, she told me that it could be a while because of the quick excretion of breastmilk by-products. She even advised me to "add a little formula after the nighttime feeding" so I could "get a little reprieve." Well, first of all, I didn't want to give my babies formula; and secondly, I didn't want to do anything that would reduce my milk supply. My babies suckled when they got hungry, which told my body to make more milk. By adding formula, my babies would suckle less, thereby telling my body to produce less milk. No thank you, Doctor!

A Routine Emerges: Starting Official Naptimes

Somewhere around five months, my babies stopped the "nurse then sleep, nurse then sleep" cycle. They had more energy, more personality, and a desire to do something other than eat and sleep. In addition to eating, sleeping, and pooping, they now wanted to play. They wanted prolonged time awake. I knew I needed to start official naptimes, but I was left in a conundrum. How do you know when to let your babies nap? How long should they nap? How many naps per day are appropriate? When should you put them down...after playing or after a feeding? Well, I decided that instead of looking this one up in the parenting section of my bookshelf, I would follow my babies' leads. And I recommend that you do the same!

My babies always woke up hungry, so I decided that my routine would include nursing first and then activity. Over time, I realized that this was a good idea because I would put my babies down for a nap awake, which forced them to learn to fall asleep on their own rather than relying on breastfeeding to get them to sleep. I also decided that I would follow their leads and tune in for sleepy cues like yawning, crankiness, rubbing of eyes, or thumb sucking. That's how I determined *when* my babies should nap.

As far as how long they should nap, I let the babies lead the way on that one too. I let them sleep as long as they wanted. As for how many naps are appropriate, "the books" say two naps per day is plenty for a six month old; however, in my experience, my babies sometimes liked a third nap too. I had two "planned" naps where they slept in their cribs. Then if they wanted to snooze on a blanket in the playroom later in the day, they could do so. This worked very well for me.

To achieve naptime success, consider the following:

✓ Nurse after your babies wake, let them play, and put them down for naps awake so they learn how to fall asleep on their own rather than on the breast.

✓ Instead of relying on time-scheduled naptimes, follow your babies sleep cues as mentioned above.

✓ You will usually notice a timeframe within which your babies will need a nap. My babies usually needed to get to their cribs for their nap within one and a half hours after waking.

✓ Always put your babies down for naps in their cribs. They will then learn to associate sleep with their cribs. Remember: Babies do best with consistency and routine since they then know what to expect.

✓ Let your babies tell you when their naptimes should be. Also let them dictate how long to nap and how many naps they need per day.

✓ After napping for a while, if one or both babies start to cry, do peek in on them to be sure they are safe. If safe, let them be for 10 minutes or so to see if they've really awakened. Sometimes they need to rearrange themselves, wake up to do so, cry for a moment, and then go back to sleep. Don't rush in to pick them up...they may not be finished napping.

✓ Be sure to keep it "day" with the lights on, shades or blinds open, and music on so that your babies know that they are taking a nap and not going to bed for the evening.

✓ Be careful with late afternoon naps, as they may affect evening sleep. (This is the reason why I let a third nap be optional and not in the cribs. And this third nap only lasted about a month or so.)

✓ Take advantage of "naptime" to get some rest, get some chores done, or talk with a friend! Naps can be great for "you" time.

The Shower Trick
In my case, my babies resisted their naps at first because they had been used to falling asleep on the breast and then getting put down while still asleep. Although it was painful to break this habit (for them and me!), I knew I had to put my babies in their cribs in an "awake" state so they could learn to fall asleep on their own. I finally began a new naptime ritual by placing them in their cribs and then walking away, but the babies started crying incessantly when I would put them down for I nap. I knew they were tired, and I wanted them to sleep. They probably even wanted to sleep! But they would just cry and cry. And what's a mom's first instinct? To go and pick them up to comfort them! This action, however, only made the crying worse when I tried to leave their room.

One especially tearful day early on in this naptime process, I decided that I would not go in to comfort the babies if they started to cry when I put them down for a nap. I wouldn't go in and pick them up, I wouldn't rock them, and I wouldn't start any bad habits. I would check on them for safety, but I would not go in. THIS WAS HARD! When the crying started, I decided that I needed to go somewhere else. I checked in...everyone was safe (just mad and crying). And then I thought, "Where can I go to get away from the tears?" because I knew the tears would make me want to comfort the crier. So, I decided to take a nice, long (okay, seven minute), shower; and by the time I got out, the crying had stopped.*

Although this may sound inhuman or terrible, it is not. It is simply an effective technique to get your babies to stop relying on your warm, soft, comforting breasts to fall asleep. It takes you and your emotions away from the crying, which allows the babies to learn to sleep on their own. And it works every time! Yes, you should absolutely be sure they are safe and not sick. But if they are otherwise trying to manipulate you, you can do your part to help them become more independent by not giving in. (*Also note that I only recommend this technique for babies older than six months.)

Starting Solids

Believe it or not, beginning solids is the start of the weaning process. I know...I know...if you love breastfeeding your twins, this is a scary thought! (If you're feeling burned out, this is a welcomed change!) But adding solids will add nutrition, thus decreasing the need for so many feedings. I will tell you this first: **You don't need to be the one to drop feedings**. Your babies will let you know which feeding they want to drop by either extending their naps or extending the amount of time between feedings. And you will enjoy not having to nurse EVERY TWO HOURS! You will still have to nurse on demand for best success. But after solids are well established, your babies will probably need less breastfeedings since they will be eating food.

When to Start Solids?

I introduced solids to my twins at five and a half months old. AAP (2004) recommends exclusive breastfeeding up until six months, and then complementary foods may be added to breastfeeding around six-months. However, AAP (2004) also states that parents may initiate solids between four and six months when the child is developmentally ready, which includes showing interest in table foods and no longer exhibiting a tongue thrust, whereby babies push anything foreign (including food if they are not ready) out of their mouths.

Since David and Julia began eyeing up our family dinner at around five and a half months, I decided to introduce solids. They didn't try to push the food out of their mouths and got the hang of it quickly, so this was the right time for us. Find a time close to six months that works for your babies! And it is perfectly fine to wait until six months old, as AAP (2004) states that breastmilk is completely adequate up until this time.

Some parents who delay the initiation of solids until well after six months may find that their babies resist solids because their flavors and textures are vastly different from breastmilk. Understanding this rationale, if you wish to wait until your babies are older than six months, speak with your pediatrician about when he or she recommends starting solids, which foods you should start, and other feeding protocols. (See Appendix B for an easy-to-read chart that includes general feeding guidelines from the AAP and other professional resources.)

For those folks who think their babies "look hungry" earlier than four months old and decide that their babies should have solids early, resist the urge! This is dangerous! As I mentioned, before four months old, babies exhibit what's called a tongue thrust, in which the tongue reflexively pushes dangerous objects out of the mouth as a protective measure. Food introduced to babies who aren't yet four months old is dangerous since babies can choke on anything thicker than breastmilk and also because solids cannot yet be digested properly by a young baby's immature digestive tract (Butte et al., 2004). Research has also shown that babies who have a strong family history of food allergies should not receive solids until six months (Butte et al., 2004). (However, please note that some pediatricians recommend rice cereal to help with reflux symptoms – speak to your pediatrician about this before adding any solids at a young age!)

How to Start Solids?
First and foremost, breastfeed first and then offer a meal of solids. In the beginning months, solids will serve to teach your babies how to eat different textures and consistencies and will provide only carbohydrates and iron. Breastmilk, on the other hand, is still the superior nutritional mainstay for babies just starting solids since it provides fluids, protein, fat, carbohydrates, and many other essential vitamins and minerals.

Regarding HOW to initiate solids, understand first that in the beginning, the main goals are to let your babies learn to eat solids and to give them the chance to taste new foods and experience different textures. AAP (2004) recommends trying one new food at a time and waiting a week between trying new foods. Some pediatricians only recommend waiting four or five days before trying a new food. Talk to your doctor about this.

There is no recommended order for foods initiation; however, many pediatricians recommend beginning with rice cereal since it is very easily digested. The cereal should be slightly thicker than breastmilk, but not too watery, as it will fall right off the spoon! Then, you could add other cereals, then vegetables, and then fruits.

You can start meats between six and nine months old, but breastmilk will continue to provide protein and fat. And your babies are also getting all the fluid they need from breastmilk too, so beginning a cup is really only useful so that they can learn to use it. I do, however, recommend beginning cups filled with water when you introduce solids since breastfed babies tend to resist anything other than the breast for drinking. They simply will need time to get used to a cup. Introducing a cup when you start solids will give them the time to learn.

In the beginning you will only need a few tablespoons of food for the whole day. Remember, they are just learning! You can start with two to three tablespoons of food with a consistency a little thicker than breastmilk (not too watery, though) for two meals a day, and work up to three meals a day. Follow your babies' leads. They will let you know if they do not want any more food by turning their heads, shutting their mouths, or crying.

Don't, I repeat, don't force food into their mouths or make them "eat the whole bowl" or you will teach your babies to overeat, which can lead to obesity! Let them lead you: They are very capable of telling you with their actions and facial expressions when they have had enough! (More on this in Chapter 20.)

Below you will find the order and duration that I followed for initiating solids. Use it only as an example, and **talk to your pediatrician about how you should initiate solids.** Also, check out Appendix B for a chart on when you should initiate certain foods based on AAP and other professional guidelines. Know that if any food causes **gas, diarrhea, vomiting, rash, runny nose, or severe irritability**, you should stop this food and retry it in two weeks or so. Call your doctor if you have any concerns, and absolutely call 911 if your baby is having difficulty breathing or other signs of a more severe reaction.

Cereals
✓ Baby rice cereal for one week.
✓ Baby barley cereal for one week.
✓ Baby oatmeal cereal for one week.

Note:
- I used prepackaged Gerber® or Beechnut® brands of cereal, which are fortified with necessary iron. If you make your own cereals, ask your pediatrician about iron drops.

- I started mixed cereal with wheat after nine months. Ask your pediatrician when you should start wheat, especially if anyone in your family has a wheat allergy or gluten intolerance (which includes sensitivity to wheat, rye, barley, and some oats since they can be contaminated with gluten) (Butte et al., 2004).

- As you add new foods, you can still use previously tried foods. When you start vegetables, for example, you can use familiar veggies with a new one. Stick with the new one for four days or so, and don't add anything new until those four (or more) days are up.

- If your baby or babies have a reaction, stop the offending food, continue to wait for the four days using previously tried foods, and then try something new. Then, you can retry the "reaction" food in two weeks or so. (Ask your pediatrician first in the event of a more severe reaction.)

- Also, the first foods you introduce should be cooked foods. (Jarred baby foods are cooked and inspected for safety.) You can later introduce raw versions of fruits and soft veggies in a mashed or pureed form around nine months old.

- Between seven to nine months old, you can also use mesh baby feeders for raw fruits and veggies, whereby babies suck the flesh through the mesh bag to reduce the risk of choking (Munchkin® brand or Baby Safe Feeder™ brand).

- Become a label reader, and peek at the ingredient list. Most baby foods now have no added sugar, salt, artificial color, or artificial flavoring. Babies have a new, fresh palate, so they don't need the additives. Stick with those foods without the extra junk. Labels should say: "peas and water" or "apples, water, and ascorbic acid (Vitamin C)."

Vegetables
✓ Yellow vegetables (sweet potatoes, squash, carrots), one at a time for four consecutive days each.
✓ Green vegetables (peas, green beans, pureed raw avocado), one at a time for four consecutive days each.

Note:
- If you are making your own veggies: beets, turnips, collard greens and spinach can be high in nitrates, which can cause "blue baby syndrome," or a problem with the babies' hemoglobin causing their oxygen supply to drop dangerously low (Baby Center, 2005).

- I didn't believe this, but it's easy to make your own veggies or fruits:
  - Make your family dinner, and leave some of the veggies aside for the babies.

- Just cook the babies' portions of veggies a little longer in the microwave with added water until you can mash them with a fork easily.
- Put them in your blender or chopper with some water, and blenderize until you reach your babies' favorite consistency.
- There's no need to add salt or sugar.
- Keep your food processor or chopper right on the counter to make this process more convenient!

Fruits
✓ Jarred fruits like applesauce, bananas, pears, and peaches, one at a time for four consecutive days each.
✓ Once you add fruits and the babies tolerate them well, add fruit when you serve cereal since the vitamin C will help increase iron absorption.
✓ To save money, you can also use adult-types of "natural" applesauce. These ingredient lists should say: "apples, water, ascorbic acid (Vitamin C)." And that's all they should say! (For example, Mussleman's® Natural Applesauce.)
✓ You can also buy the "natural applesauce cups" with added fruits like mango or peaches. Look for those that do **not** have added sugars, high fructose corn syrup, or artificial flavors or colors.

After these:
✓ You can then introduce any fruits or vegetables in any order as long as you wait four days in between starting new foods. That way, if either of your babies has a sensitivity to a certain food, you can determine which food caused the reaction.

✓ You can add meats between six and nine months. Out of convenience, you can use the jarred variety, but note that these have very little meat in them.

✓ You can also cook an extra portion of lightly seasoned meat (with a little onion powder, for example), blenderize well with water, and serve.

✓ For any foods I prepared, I measured them to equal the same volume that I usually gave from the jars. For example, if I gave a four-ounce jar of meat, I measured out four ounces or a half-cup of meat.

- 1 small jar = 4 oz. = ½ cup
- 1 cup = 8 oz. = 16 Tablespoons

✓ Even though some "Level 2 for Six Months and Older" baby foods have dairy added (milk, cheese, butter, yogurt), it is a good idea to wait until your babies are nine months or older to introduce these.

✓ For yogurt, I used those jarred varieties with the least amount of additives (Beechnut® baby yogurt) added to plain, whole milk yogurt at nine months old. (For example, 4 oz. Beechnut® yogurt added to 4 oz. of plain, whole milk yogurt.) Or, you can use plain whole milk yogurt with baby food fruit added. Ask your pediatrician when you can add yogurt.

✓ Be careful with meat dinners with noodles or egg in the ingredient list. Most pediatricians recommend waiting until one year of age before adding eggs, and my pediatrician recommended waiting until two years of age! Ask you pediatrician when it's okay to introduce eggs and egg products.

Should I Give Breastmilk or Food First?

As I've mentioned, breastmilk gives your babies their carbohydrate, protein, fat, fluid, and essential vitamins and minerals (except vitamin D, iron, and fluoride, which are in low in breastmilk). The babies' new diet of cereals, fruits, and vegetables only gives carbohydrate. Therefore, breastfeed first and then give solids.

Safety

✓ If your babies' saliva comes in contact with the food even once, the enzymes from the saliva can spoil the food. Therefore, even if the babies take one bite of a food and decide they don't want anymore, you need to throw the food out. Otherwise, they may get sick. Instead, pour smaller quantities from jars into bowls to reduce waste.

✓ Jarred baby food is good for only two days in the fridge.

✓ You can serve jarred baby foods at room temperature. For heating, follow the instructions on the jar and give the food a good, vigorous stirring to reduce the risk of burns from "hot spots."

✓ Many pediatricians recommend delaying the introduction of certain foods since they are considered allergenic or dangerous:

  – Whole milk, eggs, peanut butter, nuts, soy, raw berries, citrus fruits, fish, seafood, chocolate, honey, and corn syrup.

- Ask your pediatrician if there are others you should avoid, and be sure to mention food allergies in your family.

- See Appendix B for general nutrition guidelines for different ages and stages.

✓ AAP (2004) also recommends that solids be sufficiently mashed or pureed to reduce the risk of choking.

✓ Avoid hot dogs, raisins, raw carrots, popcorn, nuts, grapes, round candies, and other foods with a similar shape until four years of age to reduce the risk of choking (AAP, 2004).

The Procedure
To make your life easier, I first want to suggest using one bowl and one spoon for feeding both babies (unless one baby is clearly sick, then separate the food and use separate spoons). Give the babies their own sippy cups of water; but make feeding easier with one bowl and one spoon in your hand! Talk to your doctor about this if you have any reservations. But think about it: they share teething toys and sneeze on each other and breathe on each other constantly! Sharing the same food and spoon is no different!

MEAL TIME WITH TWINS IS FUN!

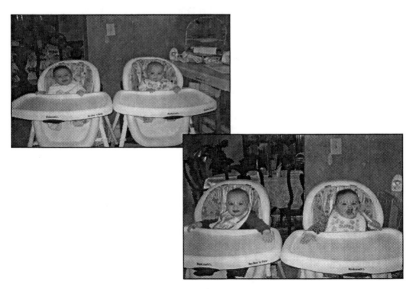

High chairs are easier on your back for feeding than the low to the ground feeding chairs. Just be sure that your babies have good head support prior to putting them in their high chairs. And **always** buckle them in and attach the tray for safety. In addition, NEVER leave the babies unattended in their high chairs!

Cups and Beverages
Your breastfed babies may need a trial of different sippy cups to see what type they prefer. They will prefer drinking from your breasts, so finding the right sippy cups will take some trial and error. Since they prefer drinking from you, it will also take some time to get your babies to accept the cup. Introduce the cup when you start solids, and be patient. They will eventually get the hang of it!

Introducing a cup at the same time you begin solids will ease them into using it, rather than having a time crunch when they turn one year of age and should start drinking whole milk from a cup. And if your babies never get bottles, introduce whole milk at one year in a cup, not in a bottle! Then you can avoid weaning from a bottle to a cup, which can be an emotional process!

When introducing cups, fill them with ONLY water or breastmilk. Don't try to get them to accept the cup more quickly by putting juice or anything sweet into the cup. According to many pediatricians and based on my training as a dietitian, juice is not necessary for your baby. In fact, there are several reasons why it is a great idea NOT to introduce juice at all.

✓ First of all, juice, even 100% juice, fills up your babies since it is simply liquid calories and liquid sugar. Instead, babies should get full on nutrition: breastmilk or solid foods.

✓ Second, juice provides no fiber, whereas the jarred fruit has fiber.

✓ Third, juice can cause dental caries (cavities) since the sugar in juice can sit on your babies' new teeth.

✓ Fourth, juice can cause obesity if your babies get used to drinking sweet beverages. Drinking sweet beverages provides extra calories, which leads to weight gain.

✓ Fifth, the acidity in juice can cause severe diaper rash!

✓ Sixth, would you put soda in your babies' sippy cup? Juice has the same sugar content as soda. (See the Nutrition section in Chapter 5.) Yes, juice has vitamin C, but so do some sodas! Give your babies the food sources of vitamin C instead. (If you feel you must add something to water to make it more interesting, add only a splash of juice to the water in the babies' cups.)

Teeth

Teeth can come in at virtually any time. Once they do, you should make it a habit of wiping them with a wet washcloth in the mornings and evenings. You do not need to use a baby toothbrush until your babies are older and have more teeth, and you don't need anything on the toothbrush but water. The main goal is to wipe off the teeth and get the babies used to tooth brushing. Also know that you do not need to use trainer toothpaste, and you shouldn't use fluoride toothpastes! Ask your pediatrician or dentist when to begin toothpastes, what types they recommend, and when the first dental visit should be scheduled.

Weird Stuff

There are some interesting facts that I discovered about foods I introduced. In fact, I wish other moms had told (or warned) me about some of these things!

Food Fact # 1: Babies love carrots. They are one of the first vegetables you should introduce, but be sure you have carpet cleaner and a laundry stain stick on hand, especially if your babies are pukers! Carrot stains are very difficult to remove, so get the big bibs out and put play clothes (or no clothes!) on the twins. If carrots get on your carpet, treat it immediately. (I have cream-colored carpet that now has swirls of orange from pureed carrot that would not come out!)

Food Fact # 2: Prunes...While great for constipation, on normal days, prunes cause MAJOR explosive poop! To start, don't give your babies more than one jar per day (for both babies to share). Otherwise, you will see more poop than you care to (through the diaper, up the back, on the clothing, etc.)! And if you happen to go anywhere on "prune" days, always bring two extra outfits! Trust me! If, on the other hand, your babies are constipated, prunes work like a charm!

Food Fact # 3: Serve avocado! Although it doesn't come in a jar, avocado is nice and plain, easy to puree, and a good source of the very nutritious monounsaturated fat. And babies love it! Just take off the skin, discard the pit, puree it in a chopper with some water, and babies will open wide for more! You just may want to puree the avocado prior to your babies being in the kitchen since the loud sound of a food processor may scare them.

Food Fact # 4: Corn should be avoided until your babies are one year old. While corn is not typically allergenic, it is very difficult to digest. Your babies will cry and likely have a lot of gas for the whole day and night after eating just a small jar of baby food corn. Take it from me, corn has its place in a ONE YEAR

OLD'S diet, not an infant's! As for the puff snacks that come in "corn" flavor, these are fine because they are so refined and the corn is so broken down that digestion is much easier on baby bellies.

When To "Drop" Feedings?

One of the main things I pondered during this timeframe was: *When should I "drop" a feeding?* In my mind, I thought that adding solids would make my babies fuller, thus decreasing the number of feedings per day. I wondered which feeding I should "drop," so I asked my pediatrician about all this.

My pediatrician told me that I shouldn't "drop" feedings or be the one to decide that my babies no longer need a particular feeding. She simply told me that my babies would tell *me* when they no longer wanted a particular feeding, or they would go longer between feedings naturally by taking longer naps or changing their schedule. That's why I recommend a routine and not a schedule with set times for set activities. Babies will generally follow the same routine, but will constantly change the times of their activities/feedings/naps/bedtime.

Let your babies guide you. Let them change their schedules according to their needs, and let them decide which feeding they no longer need. If you become frustrated that your babies aren't following an exact schedule with exact times, please know that babies are great at listening to their body clocks. Let them lead the way to schedule changes and feeding changes, and trust nature! And as always, talk to your pediatrician if you have concerns.

Physical Activity

It is also important to allow your babies to move about freely to develop properly and to meet physical developmental milestones. Butte et al. (2004) recommends limiting excessive use of infant restraints, balancing sedentary pastimes with active ones, and making a conscious effort to allow your children to move in a safe and supervised play environment. Butte et al. (2004) also makes the recommendation to avoid television for children under two years old since it may negatively affect development and decrease physical activity.

Vitamins

At six weeks old, your pediatrician may have recommended an over the counter vitamin supplement for your babies with Vitamin D and iron (e.g., Poly-Vi- Sol®) since breastmilk is a poor source of Vitamin D. At six months, ask your doctor about a change in vitamins. All baby cereals are fortified with iron, so your baby shouldn't need iron in a vitamin any longer. In addition, if your water is not fluoridated, your baby will need an over the counter vitamin with fluoride. The vitamin should also still have vitamin D since breastmilk contains low amounts.

You may be wondering, as I was, why breastfed babies need vitamins since breastmilk is so natural and what nature intended. Well, the body synthesizes vitamin D from the sun. Before the days of vitamins, moms took their babies out in the sun to attain this vitamin. Also, typically babies have iron stores from you during pregnancy to get them through until about six months, which is when it is recommended to start solids and iron sources (like iron fortified baby cereals). However, if your babies came early, they didn't have the time in utero to get all of their iron stores and thus need a vitamin with iron. (Also note: Babies receive vitamin K at birth to prevent hemorrhagic disease.)

Nursing Strikes

In my situation, the five to seven month old timeframe brought with it a new and annoying occurrence: nursing strikes. In fact, nursing strikes (not thrush or mastitis) were the only things that made me consider stopping breastfeeding since I found them so frustrating. At first, I just didn't understand nursing strikes, and I definitely did not know what to do to prevent or treat them. Here is a recap so that you can get through these with less frustration and more awareness:

Nursing Strike Symptoms:	Possible Causes:	Possible Cures:
• Refusal of the breast • Attempts to get away from you • Wants to move/play • Plays with nipple/ other body parts • Plays with sibling (pulling hair, poking eyes, etc.)	• Waiting too long to nurse • Too many distractions • New environment • New perfume or deodorant • Overtired and off routine • Hurt feelings • Mommy is on phone or talking to someone in room • Teething or getting sick • Exercising independence or trying out a new skill • Not hungry due to solid foods • Possibly time to nurse less often (Ask pediatrician how many feedings per day)	• Nurse the babies promptly or when sleepy • Limit or reduce distractions • If not home, nurse in a quiet area • Stick to your natural scent • Try to keep babies on routine • Comfort hurt feelings with love • Don't talk on the phone • Ask others for privacy and quiet • Keep illness or teething in mind and try for a better feeding later or when the babies are sleepy • Remember that nutritional needs change as babies get older and eat increased quantities of solids

As mentioned earlier, I truly believe that nursing strikes are brought on by boredom, distractions, frustration, or tiredness. See Chapter 10 for more thorough descriptions of what a nursing strike looks like, what may cause a nursing strike, and how you can overcome these frustrating moments.

A Challenging and Squirmy Time, But You CAN Continue Breastfeeding!

At this time, your babies will indeed become squirmy. They may begin rolling around or crawling like crazy, so you can expect the babies to show a decreased desire to nurse since they'd rather be exploring your home. When you add solids, your babies may also need less time suckling and may even need less breastfeedings per day. This is normal and is actually the beginning of the weaning process.

Based on my experience with squirmy five to seven month old twins, my recommendation to you is to do your best to nurse them. Your babies love you and love to breastfeed, but at times they will be preoccupied. Know that there will be great feedings and not so great feedings. This is completely normal. And at the end of the day, the babies probably will have gotten as much breastmilk as they need.

During this timeframe, one thing I found with my twins was that they would nurse together until I let down or had my milk ejection. After my let down, they would suckle happily until the milk slowed, and then one baby would sometimes become bored and start to roll around. I would then allow the bored baby to play at the side of the loveseat while the other one got a good feeding. When the fed baby finished, I would then spend some time getting some more milk into the bored baby. I only had to do this on occasion, but it worked and eased my mind that my babies were getting "enough" to drink.

Since your babies may become squirmy and may be trying to exercise their independence, I will also warn you that they may try to jump off your loveseat. This happened once with Julia and twice with David. It was scary when they threw themselves off the loveseat (Thank goodness the loveseat was low and close to the ground)! Thankfully, they were okay after their jumps, but please learn from my mistakes. **Please don't take your eyes off your babies from about four months old when using the loveseat to feed.** From four months on (or earlier for some babies!), your babies can and will fall if you don't pay full attention while utilizing your loveseat to breastfeed when you are alone. In fact, expect that they will try to do this, and you will be able to prevent a fall.

If you have a helper, you will significantly decrease the risk of falls from the loveseat. Otherwise, don't take your eyes off your babies. Keep the squirmier baby in your arms while you set your other baby down on the loveseat.

Or better yet, put the babies on the floor by the loveseat and pick them up from the floor to put them on your nursing pillow. This is the safest method (although it doesn't work once they are fast rollers or crawlers!). Do what you have to if you are nursing them alone, but put safety first! Watch them and do whatever it takes to prevent falls. (You can also place pillows on the floor for added safety.)

At this time, your babies may also begin to poke each other's eyes, ears, or mouths while nursing. They may also start to pull each other's hair or pinch you with their hands. They may even grab at your nipples! They are learning to use their hands, which eventually allows them to self-feed, but this can also become nothing short of annoying while you are trying to tandem breastfeed. My suggestion: Again, do what you have to in order to keep them nursing well.

When Julia would try to poke out David's eyes, I held my hand in between them for safety. When David would pull Julia's hair, I showed him a button on my shirt so he'd pull that instead. I've even heard of mothers wearing interesting beaded necklaces so that their babies had something with which to play while nursing. Stated simply, your babies will begin requiring more stimulation, even while nursing. Do what you can to make their breastfeeding experience more interesting and also safe.

Bedtime

For me, the seven-month mark was the beginning of difficult bedtimes. Julia fought bedtime worse than David, but there were many difficult times when both babies gave me a hard time going to sleep. All along, our sleep ritual included turning off all the lights, turning on the nightlights, getting into pajamas and fresh diapers, and nursing to sleep.

I knew that the babies needed to stop nursing to sleep; and at seven months old, both babies decided that they wanted to go to bed awake. This was great, and my husband and I would just put them down in their cribs. Typically, they would drift off to sleep like angels.

But then, Julia started having tantrums or nursing strikes because she did not want to go to sleep. She would nurse, and then bother David. Nurse, and then test me. Nurse, and then cry. Once in her crib, she'd cry some more. And I almost wanted to cry. I continued our normal sleep ritual, and I hoped for the best...that bedtime would be peaceful once again.

Although it took a few difficult weeks of bedtime troubles and a few times of missing my favorite evening television shows, persistence and time paid off. Eventually, my twins ended up sleeping 12 hours each night in addition to their two decent daytime naps!

One important point to remember regarding sleep habits and raising children in general is: **YOU, the parents, create both good and bad habits.** If you get into the habit of rocking for 20 minutes prior to bedtime, the baby will ALWAYS expect this. When trying to break the habit, you will definitely endure a good three to seven nights of hell until a new habit is formed. Always remember this simple fact, especially when you are doing something revolving around the bedtime ritual.

DAVID & JULIA, 7 MONTHS, IN THEIR CRIBS NEXT TO ONE ANOTHER

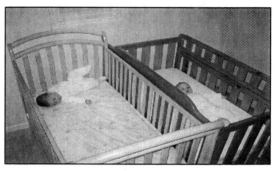

In my case, I started the bad habit of letting Julia practice sitting up in the middle of a nursing strike as David nursed with contentment on the other breast during our bedtime feeding. It kept her quiet while I nursed him, but it became a real pain despite my rock hard, left-side tricep muscle that resulted from trying to help her sit up.

Also, during the second nap of the day, David got into the habit of fighting the nap with SUCH a sad cry. He had never cried that way, so I kept going into the room to pick him up and comfort him, which of course made him cry harder when I left. So I said to myself, "Don't do it. Peek in to make sure he's safe, and then take a shower!" And sure enough, he was eventually fine after five minutes of tears. And within two days, he stopped crying at the second nap all together.

If bedtime becomes difficult, I have discovered a few ways to get your nursing strikers or bedtime-resisters to bed:

1. First and most importantly, get your twins out of the habit of nursing to sleep at bedtime. If they can get to sleep on their own at naps, then they can do the same at bedtime. Remember, it will be three to seven nights of hell until your babies get accustomed to going to bed awake, but you and the babies will get through it. And you will help your babies become more independent by getting them to sleep on their own from an "awake" state.

2. Take off your shirt. Let baby stroke your arm or warm skin for comfort while nursing. (I even did this in the wintertime.) This helps to comfort and calm your babies during their "before bed" breastfeeding session.

3. Don't engage in boisterous play prior to bedtime. Make nighttime play peaceful by reading books or by snuggling instead.

4. In much the same way, don't watch violent or loud television shows with the babies prior to their bedtime.

5. From noon on, don't eat chocolate or other caffeine-containing foods or drinks...these pass into your milk and can make the babies more active (which is NOT the thing you want at bedtime).

6. Model gentle behavior by handling your babies gingerly at the bedtime feeding.

7. If baby needs a break during this feeding or decides to go on strike, let her lay to the side of you on the loveseat. Let your other twin finish nursing and have your spouse put that twin down to sleep awake. Then you can re-focus on the striking baby and get her to nurse peacefully. Be sure to put her down awake.

8. If baby is still active and has had enough to eat, try holding her firmly with her ear against your chest. The sound of your heartbeat may comfort her.

9. Try to keep to a bedtime around the same time every night. Babies do have internal clocks and will notice drastic changes in their sleep schedules.

10. If your babies are getting extremely fussy and fight bedtime even after following the same routine as usual, they may be over tired. In this instance, you may need to begin an earlier bedtime.

11. Once you put her down, don't rush in if she starts to cry. I had the 10-15 minute rule whereby if one or both babies were still crying; I would then go in to comfort them. If both are crying, bring your spouse or a helper.

12. Don't immediately pick up your crying babies if you need to go in to calm them down. Instead, put your hand on their bellies, "shhhhhh" them, or rub their backs to get them to a calmer state. They will eventually become used

to this technique and realize that you aren't going to pick them up. And eventually, the crying will stop all together because they will know how to get themselves to sleep. (Note that sometimes they may be inconsolable, and it is okay to pick them up to comfort them in this instance.)

13. If one or both babies are sick or are in the middle of transition (moving to a new home, vacationing, etc.), forget the aforementioned techniques. Instead, try to stick to normal routine as best as possible but add extra comfort...extra snuggling, hugs and kisses, etc.

One other fact that I must mention is that your five to seven month old babies may be rolling around their cribs and may end up sleeping on their stomachs. This is okay. As long as they know how to roll and put themselves onto their tummies, there is no need to turn them over. But definitely continue to put them to sleep on their backs. As for toys, blankets, and stuffed animals: Your babies may still get caught in blankets and can still potentially get stuck headfirst in a stuffed animal, so avoid these for the time being. Ask your pediatrician when it is *completely* safe to add these.

Goal Setting

First and foremost, I am a stay-at-home mom/breastfeeding mom/author. I do not like the term my mother used for herself: "homemaker." In fact, in grade school, when asked my mother's occupation, using that term to describe my mom's job always embarrassed me. (Don't get me wrong: I'm SO glad she stayed home and truly believe that her staying at home helped shape the person I am today. I just wish the term "stay-at-home-mom" existed back then.) To clarify matters for all, I told my husband and family that my job was to care for, nurture, and grow the children, not to wear an apron and pearls and high-heels and have a five-course dinner ready by 5:30 pm.

I did like to have dinner ready as often as possible (even if it was grilled cheese and tomato soup from the can), and I liked to keep my house clean, safe, and sanitary. However, I was not obsessive about having the perfect home or making dinner every night. My job was caring for and breastfeeding two babies. (For those of you who plan on going back to work part- or full-time, attaining a perfect home or nightly dinners is even more impossible! Kudos to you for all your efforts at home, with the kids, and at work!)

During this time, I did start to settle into my role, and I felt I had a good routine going as a stay-at-home mom. I even started to notice that I had some FREE TIME on certain days or nights (when the babies would nap longer or during evening hours/post-bedtime). Being "Type A," I started planning, in my mind, a huge list of things I "should" do. And what happened next? I overwhelmed myself and caused unnecessary stress.

I decided that I needed to begin goal setting: reasonable and attainable goals with very loose timelines. I created a very loose "to-do" list with NO completion dates, and I decided that I should only attempt to tackle one project at a time and one project per day. The list also helped me to weed out unnecessary tasks or projects (for example, making cupcakes for the Easter egg hunt when I could buy them for $5.00 at the grocery store).

To illustrate my goal setting system, I decided that I would do a full house cleaning once per month (12 times a year) at the beginning of the month, and I would only spot-clean bathrooms and do vacuuming as needed in between. For house cleaning, I would clean bathrooms one day, complete dusting and sweeping another day, and finish up by mopping on another day to keep stress low and keep the focus on my real job as a mother of twin babies. Also, I decided that every Friday night was pizza night, thus eliminating the need for cooking on Fridays. In conclusion, the main reason I mention all this is to let you know that you needn't be "Superwoman." Make a goal, accomplish it, and be proud of yourself for accomplishing the goal *and* mothering twin babies!

Last, But Not Least: Breastfeeding Five to Seven Month Olds

Breastfeeding five to seven month olds is quite different than breastfeeding younger babies. Feedings may decrease to five to seven per day, and feedings may last anywhere from 10 to 25 minutes (and sometimes longer when they are thirsty or when they need comfort). As usual, follow your babies' leads, and don't set limits on the number of feedings per day or the amount of time each feeding should last. Feed on demand for best success, and know that the hardest part of breastfeeding twins is now over! You are officially an expert and only have a few months to go!

To Sum Up

To sum up, I want to share with you the top 10 things I learned during the five to seven month timeframe:

1. Just when you think you've figured out those little cuties, they go and change on you.

2. Don't get freaked out if your babies are done nursing in five to 10 minutes. They're either more efficient, satisfied sooner, bored, or requiring less breastmilk since you've added solids. They'll make up for it at other feedings if they didn't get enough at one feeding. Trust nature! (If it makes you feel better: six wet diapers per day, at least one or two poops a week, and weight gain are great indicators of growth and proper nutrition/hydration.)

3. Also, don't get freaked out by how many times your babies hit their heads on things! I remember thinking, "How many brain cells are they killing?" My babies constantly bumped into everything, but they were fine. This was just a (painful) part of exploring and learning about their environment. (Be sure to see a doctor if your baby hits her head and begins acting strangely or if you have concerns.)

4. In this timeframe, you may see some tooth buds or even teeth! But don't be too afraid! (See Chapter 9 on biting!)

5. By now, your babies also begin to talk more! And they begin to talk to each other too! Enjoy this, talk back to them, and laugh with their little giggles! They love conversation! And they will melt your heart with their sweet little voices!

6. Within the five to seven month timeframe, your babies' personalities emerge more so than ever before. You will discover that you have two tiny little individuals with funny habits or qualities that make you love them even more! Take lots of pictures!

7. By seven months, it will be hard to believe that this much time has flown by. Cherish every day with your twins! They are almost one year old already!

8. No matter how long you plan on breastfeeding your twins, you are approaching the days when breastfeeding will lessen. If you have particularly enjoyed this special bond with your babies, be sure to cherish your breastfeeding time with them as well. I remember my husband saying, "Just think how much freedom we're going to have without having to breastfeed every so many hours!" And I was just crushed to think of it! Enjoy your last months of breastfeeding your twins several times a day!

9. If, on the other hand, you sometimes feel burned out, know that you're almost there! You've gotten through the most difficult part and you're almost at that one-year mark! And if you've made it this far, you've accomplished something awesome: You've breastfed twins!

10. It was at this point in time that I realized how much my mother did for me. I took the time to thank her for all her hard work in nurturing me and in helping me to become the person I am today.

Chapter 20:
Eight to Nine Months Old

First, David and Julia's stats:

	8 months old	9 months old
David:	15 lbs. 12 oz.	16 lbs. 12 oz., 28 ¾ in.
Julia:	16 lbs. 4 oz.	16 lbs. 9 oz., 28 ½ in.

Eight to nine month old babies are smart! I remember that it was at this point in time that my twins figured out that the doctor's office was the place where they got shots. They also figured out that they should fuss before bedtime to delay the event! They also figured out that they could look at each other and make each other laugh, and that they could cry when their sibling cried. This is the time when my twins began playing together, which included stealing toys from each other, and they also seemed to be starting to form a strong relationship with each other.

This was a time of frustration for me, the breastfeeding mother. I was used to at least six feedings per day lasting up to 30 minutes, but it seemed like feedings automatically dropped to five to 10 minutes long when my babies turned eight months old. In addition, they wanted more time between feedings. One feeding was dropped naturally, which brought me to a total of five breastfeedings per day. This part was fine, but the five to 10 minute feeds made me fearful that they weren't getting enough nourishment, fat, or hydration. However, they *were* getting plenty of nutrition...they continued to grow beautifully and always had plenty of wet and dirty diapers! They were just very efficient at emptying my breasts!

Although my nutritional fears subsided, the babies started to play more aggressively at the breast. They began nipple pulling, stomach "roll" grabbing, and arm pinching at Mommy's expense. Julia would pull off the breast, roll around the loveseat, and then decide that she wanted more breastmilk. She would actually pull on my nipple like it was a rope to help get herself back onto the nursing pillow! OUCH! Also, David was getting his pincer grasp and started pinching my nipple when he got bored with feeding. One time, he pinched my nipple so hard that he squirted milk all over his face! Your nipples can get abused! Do what you can to protect them and cover them with nursing bra flaps ASAP to protect yourself from becoming a "rope" or "fun-to-pull" toy!

Enjoy using your babies' lack of "object permanence" to help protect your nipples! Object permanence is a concept that your babies don't grasp until eight months old. Lacking object permanence means your babies assume that when something is hidden, it is gone forever. When your nipples are hidden, they don't know to look for them under your bra. This is why "peek-a-boo" is such a fun game for them!

Meal Issues

Just when my frustration with breastfeeding decreased, my confusion with nutrition began. I am a Registered Dietitian, and I could not figure out how much food to give my babies, when to add more food, and how to know when my babies had enough to eat. I always nursed them first to ensure they got their hydration and fat (and superior nutrition), then I provided breakfast, lunch, and dinner meals. Around eight months, however, it appeared as though I should add a snack based on all the literature and baby magazines I was reading.

To allow you to picture my scenario: I sincerely believe in feeding babies in high chairs or other safe feeding chairs in the kitchen to prevent choking. It's also a good habit to prevent your kids from thinking that they can roam the house with food in their hands, which can lead to thoughtless "grazing" and obesity as well as a messy home. I was carrying two babies to the high chair three times per day to feed them. Adding a fourth trip to the kitchen seemed nothing short of daunting!

Well, I made the mistake of adding another "meal" to include a four-ounce jar of food plus cereal for each child. (I was somehow under the impression that I needed cereal at EVERY meal, which is not necessary.) To make things easier for you, I'll provide an example based on what I did at eight months when I finally figured out the snack issue:

✓ Nurse in the morning when the twins woke up
✓ Breakfast immediately followed - included cereal and fruit
✓ Nap - nurse upon awakening
✓ Lunch immediately followed - included vegetables and yogurt*
✓ Nap - nurse upon awakening
✓ Afternoon snack - included only fruit
✓ Nurse in the early evening and then give dinner - included cereal and vegetables
✓ Nurse before bedtime

Be sure to ask your doctor about when to add snacks and suggestions for age-appropriate, safe snacks. Contrary to what I initially thought, adding a snack was not tedious. It was another trip to the kitchen, but it was fun and quick! My other issues, however, included how much food to give and how to determine when my babies were satisfied. The nutrition textbooks in college just did not teach me this!

Here's what I learned:

✓ When I started solids at five months, I let my babies share a four-ounce jar of food and a quarter cup of cereal, two to three times a day. This was plenty when learning to use their tongues and mouths for something other than breastmilk.

✓ As they grew and got more skilled at eating, I began providing a four-ounce jar for each baby plus cereal or yogurt at the three main meals.

✓ If my babies kept opening their mouths, I kept offering food. If they showed fullness cues such as beginning to cry, shutting their lips, or turning their heads, I stopped.

✓ Don't feel that your babies need to eat all the food you provide. If you push food and keep feeding them beyond their fullness cues, they will keep eating to please you, which can lead to obesity since your babies will not know how to listen to their bodies' fullness cues.

✓ As for quantities of cereal or yogurt, my pediatrician told me that I didn't need to measure; however, I felt that I should measure an amount so as not to give them less than they typically wanted.

✓ At eight months old, I typically provided ½ - ¾ cup of cereal for the babies to share at breakfast and dinner along with their own four-ounce jar of fruit or vegetables. I also provided one cup of yogurt* to share along with their own jar of fruit or vegetables for the babies for lunch.

✓ The snack at 4:00 pm only consisted of a jar of fruit for each baby plus some "snacks" like Cheerios® or similar small "baby" appropriate puffed snacks.

✓ I also gave them puffed snacks or Cheerios® after *all meals* to help the babies learn to self-feed.

✓ I provided a Nuby® cup of water after every meal and snack to help them learn to use the cup and to help cleanse their teeth. (The spouts of Nuby® cups are the closest texture to a breast.)

A chart of my twins' typical day at eight months old:

Event	Time	What I Gave for the Meal
Breastfeed	Upon waking	5-10 minutes of nursing
Breakfast	Immediately following nursing, usually around 9:00 am	¾ cup cereal to share** + 4 oz. jar of fruit for each baby + a handful of puffed snacks + cups of water
Nap	9:30-11:30 am	N/A
Breastfeed	Upon waking from nap	5-10 minutes of nursing
Lunch	Noon	4 oz. jar of vegetables for each baby + 1 cup of yogurt* to share** + a handful of puffed snacks + cups of water **+ prescription vitamin drops**
Bath	Every other day (with a sponge bath on off days)	N/A
Nap	1:30-3:30 pm	N/A
Breastfeed	Upon waking from nap	5-10 minutes of nursing
Snack	4:00 pm	4 ounce jar of fruit for each baby + a handful of puffed snacks + cups of water
Breastfeed	(Optional) 6:00 pm	5-10 minutes
Dinner	7:00 pm	½ -¾ cup cereal to share** + 4 oz. jar of vegetables for each baby + a handful of puffed snacks + cups of water
Breastfeed/Bedtime	8:40 pm	10 minutes

*Ask your doctor when it is appropriate to start yogurt. When starting yogurt, I recommend adding baby food fruit to whole milk plain yogurt rather than using commercial baby food yogurts since these contain added sugars and other additives that your babies do not need. Or, read the label of baby food yogurts to see if they don't have too many additives. New formulations come out all the time. Nevertheless, since your babies' taste buds are a clean slate and aren't tainted by the sugars and salt to which we adults have become accustomed, go with plain versions!

** I used one bowl and two spoons or sometimes one bowl and one spoon to make life easier. When my babies got sick, I separated everything to prevent the spread of illness. Ask your doctor about this philosophy if you have any concern about sharing utensils and food. Do remember, however, that your babies are always in close proximity and probably will be sneezing on one another or sucking on the same toys regardless.

"Tricks"

During this timeframe, my babies tasted just about every variety of baby food. They also decided that they liked certain foods better than other foods. In fact, David decided that he no longer wanted to eat cereals. But as a dietitian, I knew that David needed the iron from the cereals, as it was his only iron source!

I came up with the idea of giving "tricks," whereby you give a bite of a food they really like, followed by a bite of the questionable food (like cereal, in David's case). For David, I gave a bite of cereal, and he made a face at me. Then, I provided a trick, which was typically applesauce. The trick tasted so good that he opened up very wide for the next bite, which was cereal! It worked brilliantly!

My Breastfed Babies Never Got Sick Until They Were Nine Months Old!

First off, I must say that breastfed babies get sick much less often and with a lesser severity of symptoms because of breastmilk's immune system enhancing properties (Dewey, Heinig, & Nommsen-Rivers, 1995; Beaudry, Dufour, Marcoux, 1995). In my case, I knew my babies could get sick, but I had hoped to write in this book that my breastfed babies never got sick for a whole year! Sadly, I have to say that I learned the hard way that breastfed babies could indeed get sick; however, my breastfed babies didn't get sick until they were *nine months old!*

My husband had a cold, which I contracted and then passed on to Julia. David seemed to be fine, but Julia's cold and fever and made her miserable. My treatment for her was love, acetaminophen, and a humidifier to help her breathe. Also, she refused the breast when her nostrils were clogged up, so I had to suction her nose before each breastfeeding session (which she just loved! NOT!). Julia was under control and getting better, and then three days later…

Croup

Having been in the medical world, I knew what croup was and knew what the cough sounded like: a barking seal. But when my little boy started barking, I was in complete denial. My breastfed baby COULDN'T have croup! But he did. And the emergency room was the most appropriate place for us.

To backtrack a bit, when Julia had her cold, David had been projectile vomiting for two days after each meal (but not after nursing). My husband and I thought it was strange, but we just thought he was getting a virus or some reflux symptoms again. He was otherwise acting normally. Then, two days after the vomiting started, he started barking and having difficulty breathing overnight. That night, he kept waking up and wanting comfort. I nursed him, rocked him, and held him close, but nothing could help him get back to sleep. I just knew he had croup and knew we needed to get to the Emergency Room (ER). My sister and I took both babies to the ER (in case I had to nurse). It was 8:00 am on a Monday morning and the ER was empty (which they told me was typical – Take note!). The ER doctor was walking down the hall, heard the barking, and told a medical student who was with him that Room 13 was a classic croup case. We were in Room 13. He pointed out David's stridor, or shallow breathing that causes the neck to kind of vibrate each time David would take a breath. And then he prescribed a breathing treatment with epinephrine and a steroid injection. For home, he recommended continuing the humidifier and acetaminophen or ibuprofen for a fever of 101 or greater. He also told me that Julia would get it.

Then I told him that my babies were breastfed. The physician applauded my efforts and said, "So that explains why your babies never got sick until they were nine months old!" He recommended patting my nipples gently with a warm washcloth after feedings to prevent re-infecting the babies and also feeding them with separate bowls and spoons. I had also planned on keeping their toys as sanitized as possible. Julia never did get croup. (Thank goodness!)

According to this ER physician, after the child is properly treated with medication to prevent further respiratory difficulty or pneumonia, the main issue with croup is keeping the child hydrated. The deep coughing and swelling of the larynx (voice box) can severely decrease the child's appetite and desire for fluids, so you need to make sure that your baby keeps nursing very well. One other hint the physician neglected to tell me was that a croupy kid breathes better in a hot steamy bathroom with the shower running for a while or outside in the cold (bundled, of course) for a few moments.

In summary, if your child is "barking" like a seal and you suspect that your child has croup:

✓ Call your pediatric office immediately to see what you should do (even overnight).

✓ Get your child to a hot, steamy bathroom, or you can even put him in the shower with the hot water running (but not on the child). Your child does not need to get wet; he just needs steam.

✓ Go to the emergency room if your child has labored breathing.

✓ Make sure your child is nursing and taking fluids well. If your child is not yet taking fluids from a cup well, nurse longer or more frequently as needed.

✓ If you need to plunge out boogers to help him nurse, do so regularly.

✓ If your child is vomiting his solids, decrease the amount offered and slow down the process of feeding. On the other hand, keep nursing regularly and increase nursing if needed.

✓ Wash your hands, wash the babies' hands, and keep surfaces disinfected often.

It's hard to keep your babies' germs off each other since they like to suck each other's hands, chew and touch the same toys, etc.; however, do everything on your part to keep their germs separate. For example, cover their coughs for them and then wash your hands. Despite your babies' constant germ-spreading actions, you can do much to help prevent this from spreading (separate bowls and spoons, gently cleansing your nipples, wiping eating surfaces well, and good hand washing practices).

A Strong Gag Reflex

David outgrew his 0.8 mg dosage of Zantac® well before the six-month mark; and our pediatrician told us that if he remained symptom-free, we could stop the medicine. She said that he was pretty much weaning himself off the medication as he was growing, so she said we could stop by seven or eight months as long as he continued doing well.

We stopped the Zantac® at seven months, and David did beautifully. He had no reflux symptoms at all. Then, he projectile vomited after having croup since his nasal mucus was dripping down into his throat, causing him to gag. No problem. I knew it was from the croup. But then, a week after the croup had resolved, he vomited again. And he vomited again for the next four days...

I swore David's reflux had come back. He was vomiting regularly, crying more, and grunting during meals; yet he was still opening his mouth to eat more food. I called the pediatrician; and she told me that since David probably still had mucus from being sick, he was probably vomiting from gagging on the mucus. She said that he more than likely had a *strong gag reflex* and that new textures of food may cause vomiting as well. And they did. My pediatrician said that as long as he wasn't vomiting at EVERY meal, he was fine.

A week went by, and no vomit. And then for four days straight: one forceful vomit per day. And then two weeks went by, and no vomit. Four days straight: vomit. And so on, until he got really great at chewing new textures. Then, he was fine. (See the next chapter for more on "texture troubles!")

The Best Weight Loss Plan for Mommy

If you haven't lost most of your pregnancy weight by this timeframe, you will when your babies become eight-month-old busybodies! My babies became so active that I felt like I was constantly chasing them or following them to make sure they were safe. I didn't believe in putting my babies into play yards or walkers for playtime because I wanted my babies to explore and develop their large muscle groups; therefore, I tried to make every square inch of my home childproof. However, babies learning to stand and walk will still attempt to climb onto anything, so you really need to keep a close eye on them!

Diaper changes, bathing my babies together, and getting them dressed also helped promote weight loss for me! My babies wanted to explore and use their new skills so much that all the aforementioned tasks became a huge battle! They wanted nothing to do with hygiene or clothing, so I got quite the workout when trying to complete these normal daily tasks!

Feet and Shoes

Bare feet are very important for eight to nine month old babies. If your babies are beginning to stand up, cruise, or practice walking, having bare feet is necessary for a good grip of the floor. If you are out and about, your babies should be wearing appropriate walking shoes. However, bare feet at home help your babies to feel the floor and also help to prevent slipping. Socks, on the other hand, can cause slipping, especially on tile or linoleum floors.

Two more points: First, you should now consider pajamas without feet so that you can remove socks as needed. Second, remember that your babies' shoe sizes will increase approximately every two to three months. Choose good but reasonably priced walking shoes since they might not get much wear out of them. Outlet stores are great for good walking shoe deals!

Bath Time

At about seven months old, I began bathing my babies together by myself. This was fine, until they started pulling up onto things, including the edge of the tub. For a time, I had my husband help me while bathing them together to prevent falls; however, this proved to be inconvenient for both of our schedules. I simply preferred bath time during the day. I discovered a few other tricks that may be helpful to you if you need to go at it alone for bath time with twins:

1. First, I purchased two non-skid tub mats to cover the entire surface of the tub floor to prevent slipping. I put these on when the tub was already wet so they would stick better.

TWIN BATH TIME: FUN BUT WET!

2. Also, I brought all my bath supplies to the bathroom ahead of time to include washcloths, towels (I used adult-sized towels by this time), a step mat, body wash, toys, etc. In addition, I brought wipes (poop can happen at any time), dry toys for the bathroom floor, and two clean diapers.

3. Then, I placed both babies in the tub with lots of toys and left nothing on the shelves or ledges of the tub.

4. I also very strongly told them "no-no" when standing in the tub unless I had one hand on them.

5. I decided who was less interested in a bath and washed him or her first. If the child decided to stand up, that's how I washed him. If my other child stood up in the tub while my hands were on the first child, I gave the "free-stander" a "no-no" and told him to sit down.

6. After I washed the first child, I immediately dried him and diapered him. Then, I let him play outside the tub with the dry toys so that I could freely and safely wash the second child.

7. After both kids were dried and diapered, I encouraged them to crawl out of the bathroom themselves, which greatly saved my back. I also shut the bathroom door so that I could empty the water later to prevent their fear of going down the drain. *Be sure to tightly shut the bathroom door if you do this and promptly empty the water to prevent accidental drowning.

8.   And if you have a helper, you don't have to do any of this!

Leaving the Babies with Someone Else for Bedtime

The first time I left the house before bedtime, I went to a play with my mother, sister, and sister-in-law. I had left the babies before during the day, breastfed before I left, and provided the sitter (my husband or sister or mother) with plenty of breastmilk in bottles. But bedtime is different. There's just something about bedtime...

I gave my husband the bedtime tips and told him that if all else fails, he could take off his shirt, put the Boppy® around himself, and put the babies on it to serve the bottles of breastmilk simultaneously. Simple enough...

Well, first of all, I did not enjoy myself. During the entire play, I felt guilt for abandoning my babies at bedtime. I knew that it was going to be very tearful, and I incessantly checked my cell phone. The fact is: The bedtime feeding is so much more than nutrition...it provided David and Julia with comfort and routine, safety and security, and the love and tenderness only a breastfeeding mother could provide. My husband was destined to have a rough time.

And that he did! The babies refused the bottles. They refused to even enter their room without having HUGE emotional meltdowns. In fact, my husband had to get them to sleep in the playroom and transfer them one at a time to their cribs. He consoled them as best as possible, and he finally got David into his crib, already asleep to avoid further tears. He then headed back to the playroom to rock Julia, and she went to sleep soon after. The entire episode lasted an hour and a half, and my husband kept telling me how difficult the evening was. They all survived though...and with each additional show I attended (we had season tickets to the local theatre), they did better and better.

Car Seats

A note on car seats: Babies need to be rear facing until they weigh 20 pounds AND are one year of age. The infant carrier car seats work great with twins; however, once they hit 29 inches in length, they need to move on to rear facing convertible car seats for their appropriate weights. Despite moving up to the next type of car seat, you must still face your child backwards until they are one year of age AND 20 pounds.

Sounds simple and fine, but not having carrier-type car seats with handles makes life with twins tough since that's how it's easiest to carry them! So you change car seats and look back at your "big kids" in the back seat, and then you arrive somewhere. What do you do? How do you get them inside?

Here's what I did:

✓ Use your double stroller to get them out of the car and inside.

✓ If you're going to a family member or friend's home, call them on your cell phone just as you approach the driveway to give you a hand with one baby.

✓ At a store with carts, I still used the double stroller in one hand and a cart in the other. (My arms were very buff!) This was, however, very difficult and frustrating, especially when the stroller wheels would stick. Instead, bring a helper when you can!

✓ Some stores, like SAMS Club® or grocery stores, have carts that seat two kids or carts that have a car attached with seatbelts. Use these when you can!

✓ Once you get home, first unbuckle the more active baby and pick him up. Then you can unbuckle your less active baby and pick him up with your other arm. (Yes, you need to hold two babies at once very often with twins!)

The Nine-Month Appointment

The nine-month pediatric appointment includes feeding and sleeping questions and the same normal checks for developmental issues. The doctor will often also make playtime and safety recommendations. The nine-month visit may or may not include vaccinations, but most pediatricians will check babies' iron levels at this time.

As I've mentioned before, you truly need to trust nature and trust the breastfeeding process. Although my breastfed babies looked healthy and grew well, got their vitamins regularly, and received iron through their infant cereals, I still worried about their iron test. Needless to say, both babies had normal results on their hematocrit (iron test)! All was well!

Earrings

If you have a daughter or twin daughters, it is not recommended to get their ears pierced until after they have three tetanus shots. This usually occurs by the nine-month appointment. Ask your pediatrician when it is best and safest to get ears pierced, and ask if they do it in the doctor's office. Many pediatric offices now offer ear piercing, which is a safer alternative to the typical "mall" ear piercing stores.

Before I had my baby girl's ears pierced, I also wanted to know what care would be required and what the rates of infection were. My pediatrician's office stated that infection rates are low when ears are pierced in a pediatric office compared to other piercing locations since the supplies and earrings are completely sterile and also since they are pierced by a gloved nurse. In addition, the pediatrician provided the following care tips, which also help to decrease the risk of infection:

✓ The earrings need to be turned twice per day, every morning and evening, for the first four to six weeks.

✓ The earlobes need to be cleaned daily with an antiseptic like alcohol or peroxide on a cotton swab.

✓ All family members as well as the baby girl must wash hands regularly and thoroughly.

✓ An effort needs to be made to keep the baby's hands away from her ears.

✓ The earrings should not be removed until the piercings heal, which occurs in six to eight weeks.

✓ Newly pierced ears should be protected from any potential irritants (like food or hair products, for example).

✓ Babies do best with a piercing stud since these stay secured best. Avoid hoops or expensive earrings since these can be pulled out and swallowed or lost.

✓ If persistent redness, soreness, oozing, or any other strange symptoms occur, contact a physician immediately.

✓ Keep earrings in to reduce the chance of the holes healing over.

Last, But Not Least: Breastfeeding Eight to Nine Month Olds

Breastfeeding eight to nine month olds is a breeze in that feedings decrease in quantity and in the amount of time spent feeding. Breastfeeding eight to nine months olds is difficult because they suckle, get your let-down, and then want to play, stand, jump, pinch, or something else of that sort. Feedings may decrease to three to seven per day, and feedings may last anywhere from three to 10 minutes (and sometimes longer when they are thirsty or when they need comfort). As usual, follow your babies' leads, and don't set limits on the number of feedings per day or the amount of time each feeding should last. Feed on demand for best success, and know that the one-year mark is almost here!

After one year, you can provide feedings here and there as the babies request them, begin to wean, or stick to a "morning" and "evening" breastfeeding ritual, as breastmilk after the first year becomes the "frosting" and no longer the "cake" in terms of being their sole source of nutrition. I am by no means saying that breastmilk is not still beneficial. Many studies support breastfeeding beyond the first year and into the second year for breastmilk's continued benefits. Instead, I am simply stating that your toddlers will be eating food and drinking whole milk, and breastmilk will serve to enhance immune function rather than to provide 100% of their nutrient needs. Essentially, mommy and the babies can decide which breastfeeding ritual works for them...and I always liked the "frosting" better anyway (as I continued to blissfully nurse my two year old toddlers twice per day)!

To Sum Up

To sum up, I want to share with you the top 10 things I learned during the eight to nine month timeframe:

TWINS BECOME GREAT BUDDIES!

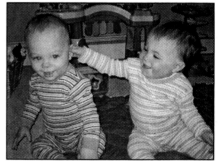

1. Babies at this age become so funny! Their personalities really shine, and you will begin to notice how distinctly different your twins are! Enjoy this time and laugh away! By the way, if you don't have a video camera, now's the time to get one! Also continue to fill those photo albums!

2. During this time, it is so neat to watch the babies' reactions to the simplest things! I once read in a magazine that what we parents consider mundane, routine, or even boring, babies consider exciting! In fact, the simplest things create millions of dendrites on babies' nerves, growing their brains and intellectual capacity! Learn from your babies and appreciate the simple things in life!

3. When your babies stand up and creep along furniture for the first time, you develop 10 more strands of gray hair!

4. I may have said this before, but I'll say it again! *Everything you say and do, your babies will say and do.* If you scream at your spouse every night over the simplest things, they will start screaming and overreacting to simple things! On the other hand, if you exhibit patience and kindness, your babies

will do the same! Basically, they are little "mini-me's" of you! Make them decent people and not monsters!

5. Some babies never crawl. They go from rolling to walking, and that is okay. Expect lots of bumps and bruises!

6. Nine-month-old babies prefer to be nude and will crawl or roll away very quickly at the sight of clothes. In addition, nine-month-old babies are squirmy and strong and will make you sweat at diaper changes.

7. Hearing "Ma Ma" for the first time truly does melt your heart!

8. Separation anxiety is real, and it can be a real deterrent to a normal bedtime routine! Stick to the same bedtime "system" and create a sense of routine so that babies know what to expect. Eventually bedtime will return to normal (whatever normal may be in your home!).

9. Twin babies always have a friend. Consider yourself lucky for yet another reason! Your babies will entertain each other, mimic each other's good (and bad, unfortunately) behaviors, and they will make each other laugh frequently. At this point, they have been learning social skills from each other from day one, so consider yourself blessed! (But it's still a good idea to get together with other kids their age too!)

10. Like your wedding day or a great vacation, enjoy every moment! Infancy flies by so quickly...before you know it, your twins will have grown up!

Chapter 21:
Ten Months to Twelve Months Old

By the ten- to twelve-month timeframe, I realized something: I have amazing breasts! In fact, I am so proud of my breastmilk! And if you get to the ten- or twelve-month mark, know that you have done an amazing job too! Be proud!

In the last few chapters, I have been providing my babies' growth stats to show what breastmilk is capable of. I hope you will be astonished at breastmilk and nature's capabilities...

To sum up, here is the WOW factor: The babies' overall stats in their first year:

The Effects of Breastmilk: David & Julia's Growth in the First Year of Life		
Age	David	Julia
Birth	4 lbs. 1 oz., 18 in.	4 lbs. 6 oz., 17 in.
1 week	3 lbs. 14 oz., 18 in.	4 lbs. 2 ¾ oz., 17 in.
2 weeks	4 lbs. 4 oz., 18 in.	4 lbs. 10 oz., 17 in.
4 weeks	4 lbs. 11 oz., 18 ½ in.	5 lbs. 8 oz. 18 ¼ in.
6 weeks	5 lbs. 15 oz., 20 in.	6 lbs. 8 oz., 20 in.
8 weeks	6 lbs. 14 oz., 20 in.	7 lbs. 4 oz., 20 in.
10 weeks	8 lbs. 0 oz., 21 ½ in.	8 lbs. 10 oz., 21 ¼ in.
4 months	11 lbs. 8 oz., 25 in.	11 lbs. 10 oz., 24 in.
5 months	12 lbs. 12 oz., 25 ½ in.	12 lbs. 12 oz., 24 in.
6 months*	14 lbs. 7 oz., 26 ½ in.	14 lbs. 5 oz., 25 ¾ in.
7 months	15 lbs. 0 oz. (no length available)	15 lbs. 15 oz. (no length available)
8 months	15 lbs. 12 oz. (no length available)	16 lbs. 4 oz. (no length available)
9 months	16 lbs. 12 oz., 28 ¾ in.	16 lbs. 9 oz., 28 ½ in.
12 months	19 lbs. 2 oz., 30 ¾ in.	19 lbs. 13 oz., 29 ½ in.

*Note: Solids were initiated at 5 ½ months.

Standing and Cruising

Although my twins began standing at nine months old, they became very skilled at cruising from one piece of furniture to another by 10 months old. In fact, by 10 months, all my babies wanted to do was climb and stand on anything and everything! This was a very unnerving time for me in that I was always afraid that someone would need stitches! Also, I had to change some of my methods of caring for the twins.

For example, I had been bathing the twins together since eight months old when they could sit up well. At 10 ½ months, however, the babies started standing in the tub. I did have a non-skid bath mat, but having two standing, slippery babies in a hard tub full of water was just asking for trouble! I decided that I should start bathing the kids at night when my husband came home from work since they kept standing up in the tub despite my constant "no-no's."

"No-No"

I also felt like I was constantly saying "no-no." I was trying to teach my babies right from wrong and safety from certain things like plants and sharp edges of furniture; however, I got to the point where I sounded like a broken record. Instead, I decided to "no-no" only big and important things like safety issues or respect of property issues, for example. And then when my babies would refrain from doing something wrong or when they would do something right, I would give a great big "Good boy/girl!" I tried to give more positive affirmations since I knew from my counseling training that positive reinforcement truly does work best.

Regarding corporal punishment and spanking: Although I am not a specialist in the field of child rearing/parenting, I have learned what works in my Master's training in Counseling. First, positive reinforcement works best. Second, what you do, your children will do. If you hit their hand or spank their butts for being mean to their sibling or for acting defiantly, you are teaching them to hit. If they bite and you bite them back, you are reinforcing the biting and causing them to bite more. Therefore, do not use corporal punishment or physical punishment because you will essentially be sending the message that they should use this type of behavior with others since "mommy/daddy" does it.

What works? For older infants and toddlers, stick with "no-no's," removing the child from the situation or removing a toy, and use positive reinforcement for good behaviors. For older toddlers and children, tried and true methods of discipline include "time outs" or counting methods (counting one to three as a warning and then the child gets a "time out"). "Time outs" need to take place away from everyone else and in a consistent location if possible (in their room, another room, etc.), and a common guideline for time spent in "time out" is one minute per year of age (for example, a two year old spends two minutes in "time out"). Children younger than 18 months should not be placed in "time outs," as they will not understand this concept. Ask your pediatrician for further guidelines on discipline.

I also like the concept of toys being put in "time out." One day, David and Julia (at 10 months old) were playing in their toy room. I had stepped out to use the bathroom, and I heard the beginnings of a rumble. I heard yelling and screaming and grunting and then crying. I rushed in to make sure that no one was hurt, and I saw Julia with a big grin and David with big tears. Julia had taken David's "light-up" toy, and David was sad. And then he was mad enough to try and get it back...another rumble! What did I do? I told them I was putting the toy in "time out" since they weren't sharing it, and no one got to play with it. And I used this strategy from there on out since it worked! Another solution for constant toy sharing troubles: Buy two of the same toy (especially if it's a cool toy)! (I even contemplated putting this fact on their first birthday party invites!)

The most important thing is to remain consistent in your discipline methods. Once you choose a discipline routine, stick to it unless it truly does not work. But remember, kids need and love structure and routine. Therefore, if your children know that they did something wrong, they will learn to know and expect the same kind of discipline.

Tantrums

What's the best way to eliminate an annoying behavior? Ignore it! The more you give attention to a bad behavior, the more the child will do it so he gets what he wants. After a few repeated tantrums and a mommy who ignores this behavior, the behavior should stop. If the child is not getting what he wants with a particular behavior, then he should stop the behavior and try something new. Use the same concept for many other behaviors such as whining, spitting, tattle tailing, and other irritating actions.

Being Equal

One personal, emotional struggle I faced was feeling the need to treat both babies equally all the time including equal number of hugs, kisses, and snuggles; equal discipline; equal love; equal amounts of praise and encouragement; equal portions of food; equal quantities of water in sippy cups...Equal everything! But in reality, it truly isn't possible to be equal all the time.

With twins, including identical twins, it is important to remember that you are dealing with two completely different people who act differently, make different choices, and have different likes and dislikes; therefore, you cannot be equal regarding every situation all the time. Instead, it is better to attempt to be as equal as possible, knowing that it all evens out in the grand scheme of things! On the other hand, of course, you should not show blatant favoritism or sexism, for that matter, toward one of your babies. (If you have boy/girl twins, sexism is having a closer relationship or preference for one baby of a particular sex because of this trait alone.) I always reminded myself on a daily basis that everything I said and did could possibly affect my babies for the rest of their lives. Therefore, you should do everything in your power to help your babies to feel safe, secure, and loved so that they can become emotionally stable adults.

Meals

Just when you think you have a good routine going, change happens. Your babies will let you know when it's time to make a change, so as always, follow their leads. At this time, your babies may want another snack, an increase in their quantity of food, less breastfeedings, more liquid in their cups, or more textures/varieties of foods. Talk to your pediatrician if you have any feeding questions or concerns.

You may have already started yogurt, and you should also have added pureed or finely chopped meats by nine months old. One thing I will mention is that between ten and twelve months old (or maybe even sooner based on your babies' preferences) you should begin adding textures and lumps slowly.

Adding More Texture

I added texture at nine months by giving hard, pinwheel-shaped baby snacks (about the size of a silver dollar) to each of my babies. Appropriately, Julia sucked at it slowly until it all dissolved. David, on the other hand, took the whole snack into his mouth and tried to swallow it. With that strong gag of his, he ended up gagging on the snack to prevent himself from choking, which led him to upchuck his whole lunch. Needless to say, we avoided those particular snacks until a little later.

After that scare, I decided on a gentler approach. I gave each baby a small and soft piece of kiwi, and again, Julia did fine but David gagged and threw up all of lunch! Even though Julia was doing fine with texture, I decided to wait a little longer on textures for both babies until they were fully ready. (With twins, it is simpler to give the same foods to both babies.)

At ten months, I gave "level three" jarred meals, which resemble vegetable soup. Again, David gagged, and Julia swallowed the liquid and left the big chunks in her mouth. Neither child spit up, but they obviously were not ready. I threw both jars into the chopper, making the meals slightly finer, and they did much better.

Although a grocery store clerk asked me why my big babies were still on pureed foods (as she scanned all 70 jars for the week) since "her seven month old was eating pizza," I knew that I, the parent, must follow the babies' leads instead of societal expectations or food company "recommendations." In fact, it wasn't until 11 months that both babies tolerated textures and chunks. And that was okay! They were still getting great nutrition from my breastmilk and pureed foods. Please know that your babies may be ready for textures and chunks sooner or later, and that is okay!

As I've mentioned, I started texture with dissolvable snacks (like Gerber® puffs snacks) at about eight months old. At 10 ½ months, I added Cheerios®. When my babies could tolerate Cheerios® and harder snacks like arrowroot cookies, I decided to re-try textured jars of food or small pieces of our dinner. (*Note, be careful with large snacks, long cookies, or biscuits, as these can definitely be choking hazards if your babies bite off a large piece and then swallow it! Always watch and stay close to your babies while giving them solids.) At this point (by 11 months old), I decided that I also needed a good technique.

My texture technique: I first gave the babies a bite of a "level two" pureed dinner, followed by a little bite of a "level three" chunky dinner. I made "level three" foods more palatable than "level two" foods by heating up the "level three" food only. I continued to alternate, pureed food and then chunky food, until they got used to "level three" foods altogether. This took a little more than a week.

I have to warn you that some "level three" foods are chunkier than others, and your babies may fight you on some of these. If your babies resist, close their mouths, turn their heads, cry, or gag, don't push these foods. Return back to pureed versions, and then try again the next day with my aforementioned technique. Also, I generally tried to keep my babies on the same foods, but know that they are two separate and different people. One baby may be ready for texture before the other, so sometimes it may be necessary to give them different things.

Bedtime

I can't lie. I know that I previously gave bedtime recommendations. I followed every one of them; and they *did* work, but I still ended up with bedtime issues around the ten month time frame, which I think were caused by some separation anxiety issues.

First note that I had no problems with naptimes. I nursed the babies, fed them their food, played with them, and then put them down for a nap. I left the room immediately, and they went to sleep after a few minutes. They had two successful naps a day, lasting one and a half to two and a half hours each, and I knew that my twins had the ability to successfully get themselves to sleep.

But I read too much in books and parenting magazines about bedtime. I read about nursing them to sleep and how that's a big "no-no." And I agreed with that one. But my babies did know how to get themselves to sleep without nursing. They did it at naptime! And I read about doing the same thing in the same order every night. And I did that too. That one was important. And I read about putting them down and then standing near the crib for a few minutes, and then moving a few steps away every couple of minutes until the babies got themselves to sleep. That one was a pain! I did this and got "trapped" in the nursery for over an hour, trying to ease my way away from the cribs!

And then, I read about the technique where you let the babies cry; and it is hypothesized that after each night, the crying will be less and less until it no longer exists. Well, I just thought that one was mean. I thought, "How could babies go to sleep so upset? It's inhumane!" During a "before bed" nursing session one night, however, my babies started standing and jumping on me and the loveseat like a jungle gym after having their fill of breastmilk. I called my husband to come into the room, and I told him that we were going to "do it like naptime." I told him, "Let's just put them down and walk out."

So we did. The babies cried! And they cried and cried and cried. Ten minutes went by, and then just one baby was crying. Another ten minutes went by, and...SILENCE. They got themselves to sleep, and my husband and I (finally) enjoyed some nighttime television together!

It's not to say that this was the end of our nighttime troubles, but it was the beginning of a new and more effective routine for the babies. And oddly, I think this change made all of us happier. Absolutely find a nighttime routine that works for you, but know that it's okay to put them down for bedtime and let them cry it out a bit. My initial guideline was that I would go in after 10-15 minutes (depending on how hard they were crying), comfort the crying baby, and then put them back down (and repeat this as needed). I also noticed that I needed to bring my spouse if both babies were crying, as you can't comfort both at once.

Over time, my babies would wake up, cry for a minute or two, and get themselves back to sleep without a problem. Or if one baby woke up crying, the other baby typically remained asleep, perhaps knowing that their sibling would do the same in a few moments too! One thing I will mention, however, is that you should go in and comfort your baby IMMEDIATELY if they are sick, scared, or in a new or different environment (like on vacation or sleeping at Grandma's house). You'll hear the difference in their cries. If they are screaming, hyperventilating, and ready to vomit, please attend to them! Use your best judgment, and always help your babies to feel safe and secure.

Nausea, Vomiting, Diarrhea, and Fever

My babies never had nausea, vomiting, diarrhea, or fever until one week before their first birthday. My husband had a terrible virus, which included one day of vomiting and eight days of diarrhea. When David woke up one night at one o'clock in the morning, I knew that the vomiting was going to start.

David vomited for 24 hours, and Julia vomited for twelve hours. Both vomited bile after they had no food left in their bellies, and then both babies wretched and dry heaved. Both children had watery and frequent diarrhea immediately after the vomiting stopped. Neither child had an appetite, and neither one could tolerate anything solid. Finally, neither Mommy nor Daddy knew what to do. Both babies were just lying there on the floor...

As usual, I called the pediatrician's office, and they told me to continue breastfeeding and breastfeed as often and as long as the babies wanted. They told me not to feed my babies solids for 24 hours, and they told me to push water in between feedings and let them rest as much as possible.

This advice was fine, but my babies were actually showing signs of hunger around lunchtime. I decided that they should try an ice pop, and I gave them water through an open cup rather than a sippy cup so that they would get more fluid. They did great with both. David did vomit a little after both breastmilk and ice pops, but it was only a tablespoon or so. So I kept giving him both breastmilk and ice pops.

Later in the day, we tried some Cheerios® and arrowroot cookies. Again, David continued to vomit a little after each bite, but then he'd return to eating after each puke. Little trooper! He wanted to eat so badly. In the evening, Julia's diarrhea worsened but her vomiting subsided. David's vomiting improved but continued, and he had no diarrhea. David (the puker) got an ice pop (for hydration), and Julia (the pooper) got rice cereal (to clog her up a bit). Then both babies breastfed for an hour before bedtime!

General Tips:

✓ Check a temperature and call your pediatrician for recommendations. You may have to take your babies in to the office.

✓ If your babies stop making tears when they cry, do not have a wet diaper for six hours, or have dryness inside their mouths, call the doctor immediately! You may need to go to the emergency room for intravenous fluids to prevent the dangerous complications of dehydration like seizures or even death.

Nausea and Vomiting:
✓ If your babies are vomiting, breastfeed often and longer to give extra fluids.
✓ Breastfeed often even if they vomit your breastmilk.
✓ Give extra water in an open cup or water bottle to get them to drink more.
✓ Pediatricians may recommend no solids for 24 hours to give the belly rest. Instead, give them water in between breastfeedings.
✓ Ask your pediatrician's office if you can give Gatorade® or Pedialyte®, ice pops, and JELL-O®.
✓ Note that Pedialyte® is very strong tasting. If your doctor's office recommends this and your babies do not like it, ask if you can use an alternative like Gatorade® or watered-down Gatorade®.
✓ Make juice or Gatorade® ice cubes to put in their cups, or make homemade ice pops out of Gatorade®!
✓ Have a puke bucket and rags or towels on hand.
✓ Your babies may be lethargic and may only want to lie down. When with you, keep them on their bellies or sides. If they become listless, call the doctor immediately.

Diarrhea:
✓ With diarrhea, one great tip from my husband's co-worker is to put two diapers on each baby, the first one being their size and second one being a size larger. This really helps prevent "blow-outs" and extra laundering of clothes and sheets.
✓ Remove the mattress pads and keep just the fitted sheet on the mattress. Then you can remove the sheets more easily for cleaning, and you can wipe the mattress directly with disinfecting wipes.
✓ Prepare to do tons of laundry!
✓ Keep shorts or pants on your babies to prevent the diarrhea from coming through too much!
✓ Use old or worn out onesies so that if they are too dirty, you can just throw them away.
✓ Use a basin of clean, soapy water for cleansing your poopy baby.
✓ When vomiting has subsided, begin solid foods that bind with BRAT in mind: (Continued, next page)

- B – Bananas – mashed or diced bananas or banana baby food
- R – Rice – baby rice cereal or baby rice cereal with bananas
- A – Applesauce
- T – Toast – give small pieces of cut up toast

✓ You can also try other dry foods like Cheerios® or arrowroot cookies. (Also, some doctors will even recommend giving normal foods as long as the babies tolerate them without vomiting.)
✓ Keep pushing fluids, as previously mentioned.
✓ Poop may start out yellow and watery, and it them may turn green and seedy. Be prepared for many colors and textures. Be sure to call the pediatrician if the stool doesn't look right or looks bloody.
✓ Signs of improvement are increased activity, better appetite, and more frequent urination.

Fever:
✓ Call the pediatrician if:
- An infant two months old or younger has a rectal temperature of 100.4 degrees Fahrenheit or higher.
- A three to six month old has a temperature of 101 degrees or higher.
- A child six months or older has a temperature of 103 degrees or higher.

✓ Ask your pediatrician what they consider fever for particular ages.
✓ Rectal temperatures are most accurate. Apply a little petroleum jelly with a cotton swab to the end of a flexible tip thermometer and insert gently about one inch or less, depending on the thermometer. This is not as bad as it sounds...I promise!
✓ Your pediatrician may also allow an axillary (armpit) or tympanic (ear) temperature reading since they can adjust these readings for accuracy.
✓ Ask your pediatrician what temperature they consider worthy of medication. Ask them for medicine and dosing recommendations.
✓ Don't use aspirin. Acetaminophen and ibuprofen are appropriate medications for lowering fevers. Your pediatrician will let you know what temperature is a true fever.
✓ Note that ibuprofen is only recommended for babies six months and older and is not recommended when the child has been vomiting or is dehydrated.
✓ Note that ibuprofen's effects last six hours while acetaminophen's effects typically last four hours.
✓ If your babies are six months or older and have fevers but are not vomiting or dehydrated, ask your pediatrician if you can use ibuprofen.

✓ At particular weights, you can switch to *children's* varieties of acetaminophen and ibuprofen. The advantage of switching is that you can purchase a larger container. Ask your pediatrician when you can do this, and ask for proper dosages based on your children's weights.

Last, But Not Least: Breastfeeding Ten to Twelve Month Olds

If you have loved breastfeeding, the ten to twelve month old timeframe can be somewhat sad. During this time, you may start to think about breastfeeding ending since your babies are approaching toddlerhood, and this may cause you to begin thinking about an impending loss. It did for me!

On the other hand, if you are feeling burnt out, the twelve month mark may feel wonderful! In this regard, although you may feel sadness or a loss involved with breastfeedings decreasing or ending, you may gain some freedom. For example, you may be able to go out with your babies for more extended periods of time without a helper. Your family/friends will be able to baby-sit for longer periods of time so you can go on a longer "date" with your spouse. Or you can finally have others put your children to bed since they won't need the nighttime feeding.

Whether you feel saddened or glad or have mixed emotions about breastfeeding decreasing dramatically or ending, know that breastfeeding your twins provided them with the best possible start in life. You gave them a very special gift that nature intended, superior nutrition and immunity, and a loving bond. Feel proud and give yourself credit...you are an amazing woman and a wonderful mother!

Feedings may decrease to two to four per day, and feedings may last anywhere from three to ten minutes (and sometimes longer when they are thirsty or when they need comfort). As usual, follow your babies' leads, and if possible, let your babies decide when they would like to stop breastfeeding.

Many moms wish to stop nursing at one year for personal reasons, and that is perfectly fine. (See Chapters 8 and 22 for weaning tips.) But don't feel like you have to wean right away. The immunological properties of breastmilk are still very powerful and helpful for older babies and toddlers as well; so if your twins want to nurse once or twice daily until they are two years old (or older), that is fine too! Don't let society pressure you into feeling like you have to stop nursing at the one-year mark!

To Sum Up

To sum up, I want to share with you the top 10 things I learned during the ten to twelve month timeframe:

1. I finally stopped my feeding logs at 10 months old when my babies only breastfed four times daily. At that point, there were no issues at all with peeing/pooping, and I could easily remember who got what breast at each feeding since there were only four per day.

2. As I've mentioned, although it was great to think about having the freedoms of life without breastfeeding, I felt great sadness and loss as the one year mark approached since I knew breastfeeding would take the back burner to actual "food!"

3. Breastfeeding created such an intense, indescribable bond, and I am so grateful that I had the courage to begin this difficult and rewarding journey.

4. I'm not sure if research exists on this topic as of yet, but I would hypothesize that breastfeeding mothers of twins have less depression and more self-esteem in parenting their twins.

5. If you are a stay-at-home mom, despite feedings decreasing or ending, you and your babies may still be in your pajamas until 2:00 pm, and that is okay.

6. Although my babies had texture issues with "level three" foods, they loved to eat paper, bugs, and grass.

7. During this timeframe, you may feel like you are doing a lot of disciplining and saying a lot of "no-no's." Don't forget to praise all your babies' accomplishments. Remember, EVERYTHING in this world is new and interesting to them, leaving a huge desire to explore, touch, poke, prod, climb, mouth, etc.!

8. Also, don't forget to laugh with your babies…they think so many things are funny, and they do so many cute and hysterical things!

9. Dance, sing, read, and snuggle with your babies! They've already grown up so quickly, and they won't be this small forever!

10. Thinking back, it may be amazing to look at all the difficulty you faced and overcame. For me, I cannot believe that my babies breastfed so much for so long. I cannot believe that MY MILK made them grow and develop and become walking, talking toddlers! Finally, I cannot believe that my time breastfeeding my twins went by so quickly...Pat yourself on the back, give credit where credit is due, and continue enjoying your babies and making precious memories!

Chapter 22:
Happy Birthday!
Nursing One Year Old Twins & Beyond

The FIRST Birthday Party!

All those parent magazines tell you to keep the first birthday party small, to barely decorate to decrease over-stimulation, and to serve a birthday cake made of carrot juice and only natural ingredients. Well, my kids' first birthday party included three-dozen balloons, lots of banners, games, 20 kids, 35 adults, and three sugary birthday cakes! (The kids each got their own small cake to smash, and everyone else shared the real cake.) The party was a success! My twins did have big, glossed over eyes, definitely appearing to take everything in, but they had such a special birthday party! And they should have! It's not every day that your twins turn ONE!

Some other neat ideas for the FIRST BIRTHDAY PARTY:

✓ I made my own invitations using an inexpensive online printer and a downloaded digital photo I had taken of my twins in their party hats.

✓ I made my own "thank you" notes ahead of time using the same photo, my own printer, and white cardstock paper.

✓ Since my twins could not eat candy due to lack of teeth, I made "candy bags" full of age-appropriate inexpensive toys instead.

✓ The best thing we did was put our new swing set together before the party! All the children had a ball outside!

✓ My husband and I wrote each baby a letter summarizing their first year, their accomplishments, their personalities, their quirks, and why we love them so much. We decided that this would be a tradition for every birthday, and we know they will enjoy and appreciate the letters when they are older.

✓ The day before the party, we made sure the kids got good naps and went to bed on time to ensure that they would be pleasant!

✓ While we bought a large, sheet cake for the 50 people coming, I asked my sister to make the two "1st birthday baby cakes." She made each cake vanilla with vanilla icing, and each cake was shaped like the number "**1**."

✓ We opened the presents after everyone left so nothing would get lost and so that cards could stay with their corresponding gift.

Whole Milk

I was still breastfeeding my babies four times a day when the babies turned one year old. This worked for my babies and me, and I truly believed in continuing breastfeeding for nutritional and health purposes. I was a stay-at-home mom, so I could do this easily. However, I did want to initiate whole milk by cup at the one-year mark.

At this time, I breastfed my babies in the morning, at noon, at four o'clock, and at bedtime. I decided that I would add cups of whole milk at the time of the least important feeding, the four o'clock feeding, and began to wean down to two feedings per day. I also decided that I would continue two feedings per day as long as my babies wanted, but within reason for me. (I didn't want to breastfeed them until they were six!)

When I first introduced whole milk, my babies were not interested at all. In fact, despite having introduced the cup at five months old, they were not fond of the cup at all by their first birthday. I will say that they went from chewing the cup to actually sucking from it, which was progress indeed! However, I was concerned that if I dropped a feeding, they still wouldn't drink from the cup and would, in turn, become dehydrated.

I decided to ask my pediatrician about all this. I asked her if continuing breastfeeding four times daily was contributing to their disinterest in the cup. I also then asked if dropping a feeding would actually make them want to drink more from the cup since they would be more thirsty. My pediatrician felt that dropping one feeding would not be harmful as long as I encouraged but not forced the cup and watched for at least six wet diapers daily. She also told me to keep the other three feedings until my babies accepted the cup more readily and proficiently. This is what I did!

The Wean

As Chapter 8 mentions, if possible, wait a few days to wean off one feeding for your babies' emotional well being and for your own comfort. Therefore, when I wanted to replace a breastfeeding with a cup of whole milk, I knew I needed to wait four days before dropping another feeding. In fact, as mentioned, I waited until my babies became really good at drinking from the cup, drinking more than the initial one or two ounces of fluid per day (like around the time of their first birthday), before dropping their third feeding!

Personally, I wanted to wean down to two feedings per day since my babies were eating well and eventually drinking well from the cup. For me, as a stay-at-home mom, I wanted to hold onto a morning and evening feeding as long as my babies wanted these. I loved the bond we had and was in no hurry to stop breastfeeding, and I knew that my breastmilk was still providing such great immunity for my toddlers!

Weaning is different for everyone, and it is absolutely dependent on your unique situation. You also need to take your babies' wants and needs into consideration. Some babies decide that they no longer want breastfeedings, while others may seem like they never want to stop. You may decide that you are ready to wean completely, or demands in life like work, another pregnancy, or other stressors may make breastfeeding difficult. As mentioned, any breastmilk you can give your twins is so beneficial. Be proud of any success you've had with breastfeeding your twins!

If one baby weans and is disinterested in breastfeeding altogether and the other baby still wants to nurse, speak with your pediatrician. I hypothesize that it could potentially damage the weaned child emotionally if you continue to nurse and therefore give more attention to the nursing child. Perhaps instead you can pump breastmilk and provide it to both babies in the cup. Either way, I strongly recommend talking to your pediatrician or a child psychologist regarding this scenario.

Breastfeeding Toddlers and Big Toddlers

At a fabulous breastfeeding training I attended, I heard the following quote by Martha Kautz, RNC, IBCLC, Program Coordinator for Breastfeeding Awareness and Support for the Pennsylvania Department of Health. She stated, "Brain growth doesn't stop after babies blow out their first candle." In fact, in most other countries throughout the world, women breastfeed babies until two to three years old on average. That said: You can breastfeed as long as both you and the babies want. Benefits don't cease after babies turn one year old.

Toddler Nutrition

I can't believe that I am admitting this to you, but I was, again, so confused with my babies nutrition at this stage despite being a Registered Dietitian! At my babies first birthday, I was giving them both textures and purees, and my babies clearly told me that they no longer wanted purees by spitting them all over me! They also rejected lumpy "level three" foods since these aren't very tasty and since these have a strange lumpy/puree consistency. I gave them iron-fortified cereal* (now mixed with WHOLE MILK instead of water) and chopped or diced fruit for breakfast, and I gave them chopped "mommy and daddy's dinner" for dinner. But I had no idea what I should provide for lunch!

*Continue using iron-fortified cereal since it is truly your children's only and best iron source unless they are eating good quantities of meats or beans. You can now make iron-fortified cereal with whole milk to add extra calories, fat, and calcium. Also, add some vitamin C foods (citrus fruits, applesauce, strawberries, pineapple, kiwi, melon, guava) to iron-containing foods to help improve iron absorption.

For lunch, I was previously giving my babies pureed vegetables and yogurt, and I wanted to retain a healthy lunch as my babies became toddlers. While I was eating my turkey sandwich, I wanted my babies to have appropriate and healthy lunch items. I DID NOT want to succumb to any of the following: fast food items, hot dogs, french fries, prepackaged and canned high sodium lunches, chicken nuggets, high sodium soups, etc. As David and Julia spit their pureed peas all over me, I was at a loss…I gave them each a saltine cracker and decided to call on my dietitian friends.

After surveying some dietitian colleagues from Pennsylvania, I compiled the following lunch ideas:

✓ Small cheese cubes or tofu cubes, cottage cheese with fruit, small pastas with spaghetti sauce, and crust-less sandwiches filled with chicken or turkey salad. (Diana L. Flinn, MA, RD, LDN) *Note: Only use mayonnaise after you've tried egg products. Ask your pediatrician when you can safely introduce eggs and egg products.

✓ Homemade vegetable or bean soups, which also freeze well for future use. (Christine Gerbstadt, MD, RD, Spokesperson for the American Dietetic Association)

✓ Grilled cheese sandwiches; macaroni and cheese with broccoli, spinach, or other cooked veggies added; boiled chicken and pork made with chicken broth; tortellini or ravioli; spaghetti and meatballs with veggies added to the sauce; and low sodium canned veggies since these are soft. (Nicole Starr, RD, LDN)

✓ Mini whole-wheat bagels, cheese sticks, and noodles/pastas. (Jessica Pellicciotta, RD, LDN)

✓ Hummus and canned rinsed beans, peas, and lentils work great too since these are easier to chew than meats. (Jan Kristensen, MS, RD, LDN)

✓ Shredded turkey and cheese in a wrap to make mini-wraps, canned fruit in light syrup, stir fry, and homemade smoothies with yogurt and fruit. Finally, kids need to have fun and share "good times" at meals while eating as a family! (Tasha Dershem, RD, LDN)

And some of my own ideas and concoctions:

✓ Yogurt – Ask your doctor if you can use containers of low-fat yogurt at this time since these are more convenient.

✓ Crackers and cheese – Babies love to pick up pieces of cheese and love to crunch on crackers!

✓ Tortillas – My babies loved soft tortillas, folded over and sliced, with guacamole or hummus inside! (We called these "crackers.")

✓ Avocado slices – Avocado has a mild taste and lovely texture that kids love! Also try guacamole!

✓ Frozen veggies – I microwaved any and all types of veggies until VERY tender, added butter, and served these as finger foods. (Nuke these with added water to make them nice and soft.)

✓ Soft raw veggies – Try cukes or zucchini with skin and seeds removed, tomato slices with seeds removed, and others.

✓ Mashed potato or sweet potato – And you can sneak other cut up veggies into these!

✓ Any fruits – Just peel off tough skins and avoid small types like grapes unless you cut them into small pieces. (I also had to peel my kids' grapes!) Also, some fruits are slippery and difficult to pick up, so you may need to help with these.

✓ Cooked meats or microwaved* lunchmeats – My kids loved small pieces of turkey, low salt ham, cut up meatballs, or chicken. (*Microwave cold lunchmeats to steaming to kill any potentially harmful bacteria like listeria.)

✓ Homemade pizza – I made my own pizza with store-bought crusts, light amounts of sauce, and shredded or sliced mozzarella cheese.

✓ Macaroni and cheese – Go for varieties with less salt or make your own. My sister-in-law, Tara, likes the variety where you add milk and butter since these are the perfect portion size for two kids! (You can use regular butter for the first year since your toddlers need the saturated fat; but at age two, switch to tub margarines.)

✓ Toast – Use whole wheat bread with 2 grams of fiber or more. Serve dry, buttered, or with jelly! (I called toast and tortillas "crackers" since they loved crackers.)

✓ Last night's dinner – Hey, why not! Cut leftovers into small pieces and let your kids feed themselves! Use a spoon to help them out in between bites!

✓ Non-fried chicken nuggets or fish sticks – You can make your own chicken nuggets with breadcrumbs or with cornflake crumbs to "oven fry" or bake these. And you can do the same to make your own fish sticks once your pediatrician okays the introduction of fish (typically at three years old)!

✓ Buttered noodles – Use butter and whole-wheat noodles for added fiber! (At age two, switch to tub margarines.)

✓ Add that cup of milk to lunch if you kids aren't getting protein (like in the above choice, buttered noodles).

✓ But remember, no more than 24 ounces of whole milk per day so that your toddlers can absorb iron. Too much milk inhibits iron absorption! (See appendix B for Nutrition Guidelines.)

✓ Also, remember that you can and should switch to low-fat or fat-free skim milk at age two unless your pediatrician recommends otherwise. Switching to lower fat dairy products can help prevent heart disease, diabetes, obesity, and other weight-related problems.

In conclusion, serve your toddlers a variety of nutritious foods. You DO NOT need to succumb to high fat, trans fat, and high sugar foods that are marketed to kids. These foods ARE NOT healthy for your children and will only lead to health problems in the future. You do not need to succumb to this harmful advertising towards small children. While having such foods once in a while as a treat is normal and harmless, providing such foods to your children everyday as toddlers will only put them on the wrong path for life.

On the other hand, providing healthy foods on a regular basis will put your child on the right nutritional path for life. And remember; don't be discouraged if one or both of your children don't like a new food the first time. Try it again and again! Sometimes it takes many repeated exposures for a child to like and accept a new food. Just keep your pantry and fridge filled with healthy choices, and you'll be doing such a wonderful thing for your children: Giving them the best and healthiest start possible. And if you've gotten through a whole year of breastfeeding twins and giving your children the best nutrition to this point, you shouldn't stop now!

Self-Feeding

My babies LOVED to feed themselves as early as 10 months old. In fact, at some meals, they fed themselves *everything* that I served. Or they would pull the spoon from my hand angrily since they wanted to do it themselves! I thought this was great, but my mother was concerned that my babies were not getting enough to eat or that they were taking too long to eat.

I asked my pediatrician, yet again, for her take on this. She responded that as long as the kids were eating the food and not throwing it on the floor, that self-feeding was fine. She said that I didn't need to give them a time limit either. If they remained interested in their food on their high chair trays at the one-hour mark, she recommended that I let them eat. However, if they were showing signs of fullness, playing with their food, or becoming frustrated, then the meal needed to end. In addition, I will add that you will still need to feed them some of their meals or parts of their meals if the foods are sloppy (like oatmeal) or slippery (like certain fruits) or if their skills are not perfect. But let them try! And give them a spoon or toddler fork to hold for practicing!

Last, But Not Least: Breastfeeding Toddlers

As mentioned, I began my twins' birthday week breastfeeding them four times daily. Then, I introduced cow's milk and discovered that they were too satisfied by my breastmilk to even try the milk. I talked with the pediatrician, dropped a feeding, and hoped that they would drink more.

And they did. It wasn't overnight, but my babies did learn to drink from the cup well. And over the course of a month, I dropped the third feeding. (My pediatrician had recommended keeping this feeding until they were taking more fluid from the cup without too much difficulty.) I decided I would hold onto the morning and evening breastfeedings as long as my babies wanted these or by two years of age.

At this point in time, you, the breastfeeding mother of twins, will know what is best for your babies, for your situation, and for yourself. Trust your instincts with weaning, and turn to your pediatrician with any questions or concerns. Also, GIVE YOURSELF SO MUCH CREDIT! You are an amazing woman who has accomplished an amazing thing by *breastfeeding twins*! As mentioned, even if you can only breastfeed your twins for a few weeks or a few months, you are providing them with precious, perfect, immune-enhancing milk. You are enhancing their quality of life and their overall physical and mental health, and you deserve all the credit in the world! Congrats!

To Sum Up

To sum up, I want to share with you the top 10 things I learned after my breastfed twin babies turned ONE:

1. Not to be gross: But once your babies start eating real food, their poop smells just like adult poop! Yuck! Be warned!

2. Just when your twins get too heavy to hold at the same time, they begin to walk!

3. Just when breastfeeding seems to get effortless, your babies near weaning!

4. If you were never a planner or a "type A" person, you may notice that you've turned into one. On the other hand, if you are "type A" to start, you may have noticed that you've mellowed out.

5. I could not have done any of this without the constant support of my husband, family, friends, and great lactation consultant!

6. I have a lot of gadgets and had a lot of ideas about life with twins that I've thrown in the trash! I really had no clue, but I can now say that I've learned so much...

7. A whole year of my life never before flew by so quickly!

8. Motherhood is such a valuable, special, precious, and personal gift...Never before have I had this much meaning or purpose in my life!

9. Twins are also a special gift. Yeah, having twins slows down every shopping trip because people want to take a look or make a comment, but what they are telling you is that you have a gift...a gift that not many people receive...two babies...two miracles!

10. Finally, breastfeeding twins was not a choice for me. It was something I had to do...something I would do...something that would be a success. And now that I've completed my task of giving my babies the best start in life, I feel such a sense of fulfillment and pride. I am so thankful for this experience in every way.

Chapter 23:
Final Words

First and foremost, I would like to show you my "before" and "after" photos of my twins, David and Julia, as testimony that you CAN breastfeed your twins and watch them thrive!

BEFORE:
Julia & David, the day they came home from the hospital, 1 week old

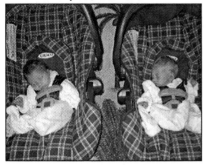

AFTER:
David & Julia on their first birthday, June 9, 2006

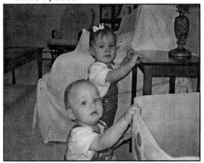

Oddly enough, I wrote this chapter right after I dumped out 25 expired jars of expensive, liquid premature infant formula. My babies were 10 months old, and I was absolutely certain that I would not need that formula "just in case" any longer. And the formula had expired, so I thought I would at least dump out the formula so that I could recycle the glass.

During my formula-dumping experience, I noticed a few things. First off, the formula smelled yucky! I smelled a milky/mineraly odor, and I was so glad that I didn't need to use it! Second, I felt great joy while dumping out those very expensive bottles of "free" formula that I got from the hospital when David and Julia were born. Dumping the formula empowered me since I knew that what I gave my babies was so much richer, so much healthier, and so much more personalized.

About that formula: You can keep it like I did for "just in case" purposes, thinking you might need it if you were ever hospitalized or something; however, please know that you were given all that free formula from the hospital to get you hooked. Formula companies, like any other companies, give free samples so that you will in turn use them and then pay big money for them after all the free stuff runs out. But here's a newsflash: Your "free stuff," your breastmilk, never runs out! Adding some formula here and there does decrease your milk supply; so keep your "free" breastmilk in good supply by avoiding using your "free formula gift" from the hospital.

If you have chosen to part-breastfeed and part-formula feed or if you were only able to breastfeed for a few months for personal reasons, know that any breastmilk for multiples is better than no breastmilk at all! Each woman's experience is unique and entails different challenges, so I will repeat that any breastmilk that you can give or have given to your babies should be applauded.

It is not an easy journey. There are lots of tears, frustrating moments, unsupportive or negative people, and things you think you'll never get through; *but you will.* Keep going. Don't stop breastfeeding your twins. Get support, get help, and surround yourself with positive people. Look at what's good, look at what works, and look at what you've already accomplished. And then you will succeed. Most difficult things in life are only temporary; so if you remind yourself that the experience will soon be over, you can get through it more easily.

Looking back, I thought Julia's nipple confusion would never end. I thought she'd never like to breastfeed. I thought I would have to give her bottles of pumped milk for the entire first year. And my greatest fear was that we wouldn't bond as we should since she was slow to taking the breast. But persistence and patience paid off. As I watch her nurse even now, she loves breastfeeding and she loves me. Our bond is indescribable, and I'm so glad I did not quit.

And then I had thrush, and then mastitis, and then the babies became active and began nursing strikes. Persistence, patience, and time...and here I am, saddened by thoughts of the babies weaning as I write this chapter. I cannot believe that my journey is almost over. While I am saddened in a way, I am so glad that I never gave up.

My ultimate advice to you is to surround yourself with support, keep a positive attitude, be persistent, be patient, and give difficult situations the time to pass...because the good stuff far outweighs the bad. And before you know it, your journey will be over too.

**Don't stop here! I've written some really cool appendices! Read on for more information on the advantages of breastfeeding for mom and babies, infant and toddler nutrition, and safe water.

Appendices

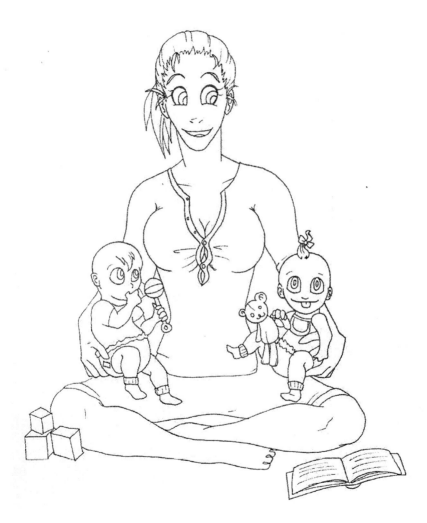

Appendix A:
Health Benefits of Breastfeeding for Babies and Mom

BENEFITS OF BREASTFEEDING	
For Babies:	**For Mom:**
• Provides optimal nutrition • Provides safe, fresh milk • Enhances immune system • Protects against infectious and non-infectious disease • Protects against allergies and intolerances • Decreases risk of diarrhea and respiratory infections • Promotes correct development of jaws, teeth, and speech patterns • Decreases risk of childhood obesity • Increases cognitive function • Reduces risk for heart disease • Increases bonding with Mom	• Promotes faster shrinking of uterus • Reduces postpartum bleeding • Decreases risk of breast and ovarian cancer • Delays menstrual cycle • Improves bone density • Decreases risk for hip fracture • Improves blood glucose in gestational diabetes • Strengthens bond with babies • Enhances self-esteem as a mother • Eliminates the need for preparing and mixing formula • Saves money not spent on formula

Source: American Dietetic Association, 2005

Appendix B:
General Nutrition Guidelines for Infants & Children

Age	Appropriate Nutrition
0 - 4 months	**All infants younger than 12 months should only receive breastmilk (or iron-containing formula).** • AAP (2004) recommends exclusive breastfeeding until 6 months, then complementary foods (solids) may be added along with breastfeeding at 6 months old. • In using bottles, caps, and equipment: These need to be sterilized in boiling water for 5 minutes before the first use. (Water used to mix formula should be boiled for 5 minutes.) • Do not heat up bottles of breastmilk (or formula) in the microwave as it heats unevenly and can cause burns; also, microwaving destroys many of the beneficial properties of breastmilk. **Proper storage and use of expressed breastmilk:** • Always wash your hands before handling pumped milk, and be sure to use clean containers. • You can freeze breastmilk in freezer bags, breastfeeding bags, or new ice cube trays that have been run through the dishwasher (each cube holds about 1 oz. of milk). • Use the rule of 5's for safety: Breastmilk is good for about 5 hours at room temperature, for about 5 days in the fridge, and for about 5 months in a deep freezer. • Thaw breastmilk by leaving it at room temperature or by placing it under warm running water or in a bowl of warm water. • Remember: Never give a bottle to help a baby to get to sleep, as it can cause baby-bottle tooth decay and ear infections.
4 - 6 months (continued next page)	**At about 4-6 months when the infant is developmentally ready, add a supplemental iron source through iron-fortified infant cereals.** • Infants will need about 1 ounce (1/2 cup) of dry infant cereal (in a bowl fed by a spoon) throughout the course of a day to meet their iron requirements. • Iron-fortified cereals should NEVER be mixed into a bottle (unless a pediatrician recommends this for reflux). • Iron-fortified rice cereal is typically the first solid food introduced, and then other cereals such as barley and oats may follow. • If you have gluten intolerance in your family, ask your pediatrician when to introduce barley and wheat. (Some pediatricians recommend waiting until 9 months old before giving wheat.)

4 - 6 months (continued from last page)	• Introduce cereals one at a time for a week, and then try a new one. • Vegetables and fruits may be introduced next, one at a time for four days before trying any new ones. You may, however, continue the ones that were previously tried and tolerated well. • Once the infants tolerate fruits well, add fruits with iron-fortified cereals since the vitamin C helps increase iron absorption. • Be sure to use a bowl instead of directly feeding from the jar as baby saliva can spoil food quickly and make infants sick. • Opened jars of food only last refrigerated for 2-3 days. • Foods should be cooked until 9 months or when your pediatrician recommends raw fruits and veggies. • Start the cup filled with water, not juice, when you start solids. (Juice is not necessary and can cause fullness, cavities, diaper rash, and obesity. If you still want to add some juice, wait until 8 months, add only a splash of juice to water, and limit the quantity of juice to 4 oz. total per day.)
6 - 8 months	**At 6-8 months, infant foods should be strained or finely chopped.** • Finger foods like baby cereal puffs, arrowroot crackers (broken up), or dry whole-wheat toast/bagels may be added when the infant exhibits the palmer grasp. *ALWAYS watch your babies when giving these foods to prevent choking. • If given the okay by your pediatrician, wheat can be tried at the end of this timeframe (in mixed cereals, crackers, cream of wheat, etc.)
9 - 12 months	**At 9-12 months, table foods may be added to include chopped, well-cooked foods.** • At this time, pureed meats or jarred meals with meat may be offered, and small finger foods (e.g., Cheerios®) may be added as infants exhibit a pincer grasp. • "Meats" can include chicken, turkey, beef, pork, and mashed beans. Wait until age two to introduce eggs and age three to give fish. • Yogurt may be added. You can use whole milk plain yogurt mixed with pureed baby fruit, which is cheaper and has less sugar than the pre-packaged baby yogurt. • At this point, you can also add harder to digest foods like mashed or pureed corn, broccoli, cauliflower, creamed spinach, etc.
1 year (continued next page)	**At 1 year, whole milk may be introduced.** • Children ages one to five should consume no more than 24 ounces of cow's milk, goat's milk, or soy milk per day since too much milk may inhibit iron absorption. • Generally, raw berries, citrus fruits, and dairy may be introduced after age 1 since these foods are highly allergenic. (And strawberries may cause diaper rash due to their acidity even after the first birthday. Ask your pediatrician about these.)

1 year (continued from last page)	• Honey and corn syrup should be avoided until after age 1 since they may cause botulism. • At this time, you can add baked goods made with eggs, but wait on serving plain eggs until age 2 to reduce the risk of an allergy. *** Check with the child's physician first about introducing new foods, as he or she may advise otherwise based on family history of allergies.**
2 years	**At age 2, switch your toddlers (and whole family) to 1% low-fat or fat-free skim milk.** • AAP (2007) recommends the switch to 1 % low-fat or fat-free skim milk to reduce the risk of heart disease, diabetes, and obesity. • At this point, you can introduce **eggs**.
3 years	**At age 3:** • Generally, **fish and seafood** including **salmon** may be introduced at age 3. (Check with pediatrician first.) And introduce salmon now, as it has tremendous health benefits for the entire family! • Remember, it can take many trials of new foods to get children to accept them, so don't give up after one failed attempt. • Generally, **peanuts, peanut butter, tree nuts, and other nut butters** may be added at age 3. (Check with pediatrician first, especially if there is a family history of allergies.)
4 years	**These foods can cause an infant or toddler to choke, but under supervision, these may be added at 4 years old:** • Popcorn, whole grapes, whole beans, nuts, hard candies, jelly beans, raw carrots and celery, seeds, cherry tomatoes, hot dog slices (in moderation or low-fat versions), other foods similar in size and shape, and large chunks of food.

Sources: AAP, 2004; AAP, 2007; Fiocchi et al., 2006; Fitch, 2004.

Appendix C:
Safe Water — For You & Your Babies

When I began giving rice cereal at five and a half months, I didn't have enough breastmilk on hand to mix with the cereal. My pediatrician said that I could use water instead, so I went home and mixed up some cereal with my well water. Being a registered dietitian, I later thought about what I had done, and tremendous guilt and fear came over me! *What had I just done?* I truly didn't know what was in my well water, and I surely didn't want to harm my babies!

I did some digging around. Well water, even if tested regularly (say, once a month), can have any types of pesticides, bacteria, coliform bacteria (poop), minerals, or other harmful contaminants at any given time; therefore, it is now recommended by many health authorities that well water not be drunk at all by any household members. In fact, if you live near farms, you may have high levels of nitrates from soil run-off, which is known to cause "blue baby syndrome," whereby babies' hemoglobin is affected (their oxygen supply can drop dangerously low, causing them to appear blue) (Baby Center, 2005).

Well water, however, may be used for cooking, showering, laundry, washing dishes, etc. But it is still a good idea to have it tested every six months to a year regardless of whether or not you drink it. Baby Center (2005) recommends testing well water once yearly for nitrates, coliform bacteria, total dissolved solids, and pH; and they recommend testing water every three years for chloride, iron, sulfate, manganese, hardness, and corrosion. Depending on where you live, you may also need to check yearly for lead, copper, arsenic, radon, pesticides, and other potential contaminants (Baby Center, 2005).

Tap water, on the other hand, can contain disinfection byproducts, turbidity, lead, arsenic, and parasites in small but detectable amounts (Center for Science in the Public Interest, 2000). Therefore, you may conclude it's best to drink bottled water. But then again, not all bottled water is created equal. See the chart on page 239 for a better understanding of all the types of bottled waters. I chose to purchase *spring water* for my water cooler, and I felt this was the safest and best choice for my family.

In addition, regardless of what type of water you have, if your water smells funny or looks strange (for example, a sulfur smell or a greasy appearance), don't drink or use it (Baby Center, 2005). But not all contaminants smell or change the appearance of your water. You can have city tap water or well water tested if you suspect anything is wrong with your water.

What about filters? While filters remove lead and some contaminants, they do not remove *all* potential contaminants (Baby Center, 2005). Therefore, you can do one of two things:

✓ Either find out what contaminants your water contains by having it tested, or go to the NSF International Website (www.nsf.org) for a listing of the types of filters that take away your specific contaminants (Baby Center, 2005).

✓ Or call local spring water companies. Ask for a current hard copy listing of what their water contains (which should include no additives), and ask how often they test. Ask about nitrates and fluoride, and then make your choice as to which water company to use. You may need to ask for a manager or owner to get this information. (Because water filters can be expensive to replace and it would be hard to tell how long filters will last since breastfeeding moms drink so much water, I chose to use water from a spring.)

Fluoride
Also note that your tap water may be fluoridated or your well may contain fluoride from the soil. Call your health department if you are not sure if your water contains fluoride, or have your well tested for fluoride. If your water does contain fluoride, your babies and children would get some fluoride from cooking. In addition, older children get fluoride from toothpaste and mouth rinses.

Talk to your pediatrician about fluoride. If you are going to purchase and use spring water (which should not have anything added – ask the company), your pediatrician will probably prescribe a vitamin with fluoride at about six months old. While fluoride is very necessary and important for healthy development of teeth and bone, too much fluoride is not a good thing, as it may cause fluorosis, or mottling (white marks) of the teeth. You won't need to purchase the "baby water," or water with added fluoride, for your babies' cups or for mixing up your babies' food if your babies are getting a vitamin with added fluoride.

See the next page for an easy-to-use chart describing the types of bottled water and a description of each.

You can also go to the website for the International Bottled Water Association (IBWA) at: www.bottledwater.org. IBWA often completes unannounced inspections to see which water companies are compliant, and they list these companies on their Website (Center for Science in the Public Interest, 2000).

What's in My Bottled Water?
A Thorough Description of Waters Available on the Market

Type of Bottled Water	Description
Spring Water	-Flows naturally from the earth's surface -75% of bottled water in the U.S. is from a spring -Springs are supposed to be protected from pollution by industry guidelines and state laws
Mineral Water	-Spring water with added dissolved minerals (like magnesium and calcium) -Minerals added should be at least 250 mg of dissolved minerals per liter
Sparkling Water	-Spring water with carbon dioxide gas added
Drinking Water	-City water or tap water -The label usually states which city the water came from unless it has been filtered or disinfected -Examples are PepsiCo's® Aquafina® or Coca-Cola's® Dasani®
Purified Water	-Treated with distillation, ion exchange, reverse osmosis, or another process
Distilled Water	-Comes from the steam of city water that has been boiled -This process gets rid of most contaminants except benzene, chlorine, and some other volatile organic chemicals -Ask your children's pediatrician if distilled water is appropriate if you typically use this type in your home

Source: Center for Science in the Public Interest, 2000

References

American Academy of Pediatrics. (2004). *Pediatric nutrition handbook* (5th ed.). Washington, DC: American Academy of Pediatrics.

American Academy of Pediatrics. (2006). Media guidelines for parents. Retrieved June 22, 2006 from http://www.aap.org/pubed/ZZGVL4PQ7C.htm?&sub_cat=17.

American Academy of Pediatrics. (2007). Nutrition issue card. Retrieved March 5, 2007 from http://www.aap.org/moc/pressroom/nutrition.htm.

American Dietetic Association. (2005). Position of the American Dietetic Association: Promoting and supporting breastfeeding. *Journal of the American Dietetic Association, 105*, 810-818.

Baby Center. (2005). How to tell if your water is safe. Retrieved December 6, 2005 from http://www.babycenter.com/refcap/baby/babysafety/469.html.

Beaudry, M., Dufour, R., & Marcoux, S. (2005). Relation between infant feeding and infection during the first six months of life. *Journal of Pediatrics, 126*, 191-197.

Butte, N., Cobb, K., Dwyer, J., Graney, L., Heird, W., & Rickard, K. (2004). The start healthy feeding guidelines for infants and toddlers. *Journal of the American Dietetic Association, 104*(3), 442-454.

Center for Science in the Public Interest. (2000). Water, water, everywhere. *Nutrition Action Healthletter.* Retrieved January 9, 2006 from http://www.cspinet.org/nah/water/.

Charpak, N., Ruiz-Pelaez, J. G., Figueroa de C. Z., & Charpak, Y. (1997). Kangaroo mother versus traditional care for newborn infants less than or equal to 2000 grams: A randomized, controlled trial. *Pediatrics, 100*(4), 682-688.

Dewey, K. G., Heinig, M. J., & Nommsen-Rivers, L. A. (1995). Differences in morbidity between breast-fed and formula-fed infants. *Journal of Pediatrics, 126*, 696-702.

Fiocchi, A., Assa'ad, A., & Bahna, S. (2006). Food allergy and the introduction of solid foods to infants: A consensus document. Adverse reactions to Foods Committee, American College of Allergy, Asthma and Immunology. *Annals of Allergy, Asthma, & Immunology, 97*(1), 10-20.

Fitch, C. (2004). Preventing iron deficiency in infants and toddlers. *Today's Dietitian,* 6(12), 32-34.

Food and Nutrition Board, Institute of Medicine, National Academies. (2004). Dietary reference intakes (DRIs): Recommended intakes for individuals. *DRI Reports.* Retrieved February 12, 2007 from http://www.iom.edu/Object.File/Master/21/372/0.pdf.

Heinig, M. J., & Dewey, K. G. (1997). Health advantages of breastfeeding for mothers: A critical review. *Nutrition Research Reviews, 10,* 35-56.

Klaus, M. (1998). Mother and infant: Early emotional ties. *Pediatrics 102*(5), 1255-1246.

Martin, J. A., Hamilton, B. E., Sutton, P. D., Ventura, S. J., Menacker, F., & Munson, M. L. (2005). Births: Final data for 2003. *National Vital Statistics Reports, 54*(2), 1-116. Retrieved February 22, 2006 from http://www.cdc.gov/nchs/data/nvsr/nvsr54/nvsr54_02.pdf.

Mead Johnson & Co.® (2004). *Why DHA?* Retrieved April 4, 2006 from http://www.expectalipil.com/whydha.html.

Newcomb, P. A., Storer, B. E., Longnecker, M. P., Mittendorf, R., Greenberg, E. R., Clapp, R. W., Burke, K. P., Willett, S. C., & MacMahon, B. (1994). Lactation and a reduced risk of premenopausal breast cancer. *New England Journal of Medicine, 330,* 81-87.

Ramsay, D. T., Kent, J. C., Hartmann, R. A., & Hartmann, P. E. (2005). Anatomy of the lactating human breast redefined with ultrasound imaging. *Journal of Anatomy, 206*(6), 525-534.

Rosenthal, M. S. & Arsenault, G. (2001). *The breastfeeding sourcebook.* Retrieved March 20, 2006 from http://www.webmd.com/content/article/87/99604.htm, http://www.webmd.com/content/article/87/99606.htm, http://www.webmd.com/content/article/87/99607.htm, http://www.webmd.com/content/article/87/99609.htm, & http://www.webmd.com/content/article/87/99611.htm.

Tessier, R., Cristo, M., Valez, S., Giron, M., Figueroa de Calume, Z., Ruiz-Palaez, J. G., Charpak, Y., & Charpak, N. (1998). Kangaroo mother care and the bonding hypothesis. *Pediatrics, 102*(2), e17. Retrieved March 2, 2006 from http://pediatrics.aappublications.org/cgi/content/full/102/2/e17.

The National Women's Health Information Center. (2006). *Coping with breastfeeding challenges.* Retrieved March 13, 2006, from http://www.4woman.gov/Breastfeeding/index.cfm?page229.

USDA. (2006). *MyPyramid results downloads.* Retrieved March 3, 2007 from http://www.mypyramid.gov/downloads/results/results_3000_18.pdf.

Witt, C. L. (2006). *How should we implement safe sleeping recommendations in the NICU setting?* Retrieved June 6, 2007 from http://www.medscape.com/viewarticle/532685.

World Health Organization. (2006). *World health organization releases new child growth standards.* Retrieved June 14, 2006 from http://www.who.int/mediacentre/news/releases/2006/pr21/en/index.html.

Index

Printed in the United States
116580LV00003B/94-102/A